CURING COUGHS, COLDS AND FLU –
THE DRUG-FREE WAY

MARGARET HILLS, SRN, trained as a nurse at St Stephen's Hospital in London, until her training was cut short by crippling heart disease and arthritis. Against all the odds she fought back, and went on to marry, have eight children and continue a long career as an industrial nurse. She now shares her radical new treatment for arthritis through her clinic in Coventry. She has written several best-selling books based on her experience; *Curing Arthritis – The Drug-Free Way*, *Curing Arthritis Cookbook*, and *Curing Illness – the Drug-Free Way*, all published by Sheldon Press.

Overcoming Common Problems Series

Feverfew
A traditional herbal remedy for migraine
and arthritis
DR STEWART JOHNSON

Fight Your Phobia and Win
DAVID LEWIS

Getting Along with People
DIANNE DOUBTFIRE

Goodbye Backache
DR DAVID IMRIE WITH COLLEEN
DIMSON

Helping Children Cope with Divorce
ROSEMARY WELLS

Helping Children Cope with Grief
ROSEMARY WELLS

How to be a Successful Secretary
SUE DYSON AND STEPHEN HOARE

How to Be Your Own Best Friend
DR PAUL HAUCK

How to Control your Drinking
DRS W. MILLER AND R. MUNOZ

How to Cope with Stress
DR PETER TYRER

How to Cope with your Child's Allergies
DR PAUL CARSON

**How to Cope with Tinnitus and Hearing
Loss**
DR ROBERT YOUNGSON

How to Cure Your Ulcer
ANNE CHARLISH AND DR BRIAN
GAZZARD

How to Do What You Want to Do
DR PAUL HAUCK

How to Enjoy Your Old Age
DR B. F. SKINNER AND M. E.
VAUGHAN

How to Improve Your Confidence
DR KENNETH HAMBLY

How to Interview and Be Interviewed
MICHELE BROWN AND GYLES
BRANDRETH

How to Love a Difficult Man
NANCY GOOD

How to Love and be Loved
DR PAUL HAUCK
How to Make Successful Decisions
ALISON HARDINGHAM

How to Move House Successfully
ANNE CHARLISH

How to Pass Your Driving Test
DONALD RIDLAND

How to Say No to Alcohol
KEITH McNEILL

How to Spot Your Child's Potential
CECILE DROUIN AND ALAIN DUBOS

How to Stand up for Yourself
DR PAUL HAUCK

**How to Start a Conversation and Make
Friends**
DON GABOR

How to Stop Feeling Guilty
DR VERNON COLEMAN

How to Stop Smoking
GEORGE TARGET

How to Stop Taking Tranquillisers
DR PETER TYRER

Hysterectomy
SUZIE HAYMAN

If Your Child is Diabetic
JOANNE ELLIOTT

Jealousy
DR PAUL HAUCK

Learning to Live with Multiple Sclerosis
DR ROBERT POVEY, ROBIN DOWIE
AND GILLIAN PRETT

Living Alone – A Woman's Guide
LIZ McNEILL TAYLOR

Living with Grief
DR TONY LAKE

Overcoming Common Problems Series

The ABC of Eating
Coping with anorexia, bulimia and
compulsive eating
JOY MELVILLE

Beating the Blues
SUSAN TANNER AND JILLIAN
BALL

Beating Job Burnout
DR DONALD SCOTT

Being the Boss
STEPHEN FITZSIMON

Birth Over Thirty
SHEILA KITZINGER

Body Language
How to read others' thoughts by their
gestures
ALLAN PEASE

Bodypower
DR VERNON COLEMAN

Calm Down
How to cope with frustration and anger
DR PAUL HAUCK

Comfort for Depression
JANET HORWOOD

Common Childhood Illnesses
DR PATRICIA GILBERT

Complete Public Speaker
GYLES BRANDRETH

Coping with Anxiety and Depression
SHIRLEY TRICKETT

Coping with Depression and Elation
DR PATRICK McKEON

Coping with Stress
DR GEORGIA WITKIN-LANOIL

Coping with Suicide
DR DONALD SCOTT

Coping with Thrush
CAROLINE CLAYTON

**Coping Successfully with Your Child's
Asthma**
DR PAUL CARSON

**Coping Successfully with Your Child's Skin
Problems**
DR PAUL CARSON

**Coping Successfully with Your Hyperactive
Child**
DR PAUL CARSON

Coping Successfully with Your Irritable Bowel
ROSEMARY NICOL

Curing Arthritis Diet Book
MARGARET HILLS

Curing Arthritis – The Drug-free Way
MARGARET HILLS

**Curing Coughs, Colds and Flu – the
Drug-free Way**
MARGARET HILLS

Curing Illness – The Drug-free Way
MARGARET HILLS

Depression
DR PAUL HAUCK

Divorce and Separation
ANGELA WILLANS

The Dr Moerman Cancer Diet
RUTH JOCHEMS

The Epilepsy Handbook
SHELAGH McGOVERN

**Everything You Need to Know about
Adoption**
MAGGIE JONES

**Everything You Need to Know about
Contact Lenses**
DR ROBERT YOUNGSON

**Everything You Need to Know about Your
Eyes**
DR ROBERT YOUNGSON

**Everything You Need to Know about the
Pill**
WENDY COOPER AND TOM SMITH

Everything You Need to Know about Shingles
DR ROBERT YOUNGSON

Family First Aid and Emergency Handbook
DR ANDREW STANWAY

Overcoming Common Problems Series

Living Through Personal Crisis
ANN KAISER STEARNS
Living with High Blood Pressure
DR TOM SMITH

Loneliness
DR TONY LAKE

Making Marriage Work
DR PAUL HAUCK

Making the Most of Loving
GILL COX AND SHEILA DAINOW

Making the Most of Yourself
GILL COX AND SHEILA DAINOW

Managing Two Careers
How to survive as a working mother
PATRICIA O'BRIEN

Meeting People is Fun
How to overcome shyness
DR PHYLLIS SHAW

The Nervous Person's Companion
DR KENNETH HAMBLY

Overcoming Fears and Phobias
DR TONY WHITEHEAD

Overcoming Shyness
A woman's guide
DIANNE DOUBTFIRE

Overcoming Stress
DR VERNON COLEMAN

Overcoming Tension
DR KENNETH HAMBLY

Overcoming Your Nerves
DR TONY LAKE

The Parkinson's Disease Handbook
DR RICHARD GODWIN-AUSTEN

Say When!
Everything a woman needs to know about
alcohol and drinking problems
ROSEMARY KENT
Self-Help for your Arthritis
EDNA PEMBLE

Sleep Like a Dream – The Drug-Free Way
ROSEMARY NICOL

Solving your Personal Problems
PETER HONEY

Someone to Love
How to find romance in the personal columns
MARGARET NELSON

A Step-Parent's Handbook
KATE RAPHAEL

Stress and your Stomach
DR VERNON COLEMAN

Trying to Have a Baby?
Overcoming infertility and child loss
MAGGIE JONES

What Everyone Should Know about Drugs
KENNETH LEECH

Why Be Afraid?
How to overcome your fears
DR PAUL HAUCK

Women and Depression
A practical self-help guide
DEIDRE SANDERS

You and Your Varicose Veins
DR PATRICIA GILBERT

Your Arthritic Hip and You
GEORGE TARGET

Overcoming Common Problems

CURING COUGHS, COLDS AND FLU – THE DRUG-FREE WAY

Margaret Hills, SRN

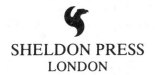

SHELDON PRESS
LONDON

First published in Great Britain in 1988 by
Sheldon Press, SPCK, Marylebone Road, London NW1 4DU

Second impression 1989

British Library Cataloguing in Publication Data

Hills, Margaret
    Curing coughs, colds and flu: the drug-
    free way.—(Overcoming common problems).
    1. Man. Colds. Natural remedies
    I. Title   II. Series
    616.2'05068'8

    ISBN 0–85969–578–6

Photoset by Deltatype Ltd, Ellesmere Port
Printed in Great Britain by
Richard Clay Ltd, Bungay, Suffolk

For my children, Michael, Christine, Graham, Sally, Clive, Peter, Bill and Mary; and also for my grandchildren – John, Claire, Richard, Jennifer, Daniel, Tracey, Julia and Alexandra.

My special thanks go to my daughter
Mary, for typing this book.

Contents

Foreword   1

1   What is Health?   5

2   What Causes Illness?   11

3   You are What You Eat   15

4   How Your Body Fights Illness   27

5   How to Cure a Cold   35

6   How to Cure Coughs   47

7   How to Cure Flu   60

8   How to Keep Children Healthy   67

9   How to Stay Healthy as You Grow Older   77

10 The Value of Vitamins   94

11 Stress and Your Health   104

    Index   109

Foreword

There are many people today who have little faith in modern medicine, and many family doctors are becoming more and more reluctant to churn out prescription after prescription because, having devoted years to doing just this, they realize now that the side-effects of the drugs they prescribe can be far more serious than the complaint the drug is prescribed for.

We can classify the side-effects of drugs under three headings:–

i   Those that cause immediate side effects.
ii   Those that have delayed reaction.
iii The drugs that suppress illness in the body, giving immediate relief which is very short lived. These do a lot of damage to the system, giving the self-healing powers of the body no chance to work.

I feel very strongly that the drug side of medicine has sadly let down the medical profession, because it is only the medically trained that can mend a broken leg, do a replacement heart valve operation, or carry out any of the other treatments which doctors and surgeons can use to save lives.

First of all we consider the drugs that cause immediate side-effects. These are really the less dangerous types – they cause immediate rashes or swellings that are quite obvious both to the patient and the doctor and are discontinued at once, and another mode of treatment is adopted. Secondly, we have the drugs that have delayed side-effects. These are far more dangerous, and when after some time the side-effects make themselves known it is too late – the damage has been done. I have found that the drugs made to relieve arthritis are the most dangerous, where side-effects are concerned – the steroids do so much damage, such as nausea, vomiting, ulceration, swellings and much more less obvious damage.

Antibiotics, too, are not very desirable – the word 'anti-biotic' means 'anti-life'. They are given with very good intentions – to kill the offending virus – but in doing so they kill the friendly bacteria that normally inhabit the bowel, for example, and produce candida infections which are extremely difficult to cure and can make the patient very miserable and uncomfortable for a very long time. These are only two of the many examples of drug side-effects which abound in the course of medical treatment.

Then there is the third kind of drug – the suppressive type. The best example here is when an antibiotic is given for an attack of influenza. Influenza is a condition that arises in the body when there is a lot of toxic acid to be eliminated. The patient develops a temperature, with a lot of aches and pains, coughing and sneezing, and all this is an attempt by the body to get rid of those toxic acids. By far the most effective cure is bed-rest, fasting and hot lemon and honey drinks – in other words assisting the body to eliminate those acids naturally. Instead of adopting this natural regime a lot of people call in the doctor, and he'll probably give an antibiotic to get the temperature down and put a stop to those aches and pains.

In twenty-four hours the patient feels better – magic! In a day or two he is up and about – but, how sad – he is still the possessor of a body full of acid that will succumb again to the slightest infection. Not only that but now he is having to deal with the side-effects of that antibiotic. His general health is very poor and he has probably got a candida infection – thrush, mouth ulcers or intestinal disturbances of some sort. If he had adopted the former method of treatment and allowed a natural elimination to take place, it would have taken longer, but the benefits would have been well worth waiting for. He would now be clean of those toxic acids – the body would be in a clean condition, his feeling of health and vitality would be second to none, and of course he would not have to cope with the uncomfortable drug side-effects.

I feel that patients need to be educated, and indeed told by their consultants and GPs about the toxicity of drugs they are about to be prescribed – they should have a thorough knowledge of the risks as well as the benefits and then be allowed to make up their own minds. After all, it is their body, mind and spirit that is being treated, and they should captain their own ship, and be responsible for steering it safely to the harbour at three score years and ten.

Unfortunately, what the medical profession terms cure is the suppression of symptoms into the system, which only causes further serious disease later. Disease, or dis-ease of the body, is nature's attempt to eliminate acids – nature's attempt at self-healing, and it should never be suppressed but gently encouraged. A tremendous amount of ignorance exists in patients' minds as to what course of treatment to follow and this is not to be wondered at, when we have the orthodox medical profession telling them that disease is something that happens to the body and they have to pull out all the stops to wage war on it, kill it, suppress it, fight it.

On the other hand, we have a second body of people – the alternative, complementary people claiming that disease is the direct result of self-indulgence, wrong living and wrong feeding. I am a State Registered Nurse, trained to believe in orthodox medicine and all it stands for, but I bless the day I was forced to realize that my thinking was all wrong – and it's strange to admit that my training as a nurse helped me to realize it. I have the utmost respect and admiration for the medical profession. They are a hard-working, caring body of people who can be called upon at any time, day or night, and can be relied upon to give cheerful, helpful service. Their responsibility is great, carrying the weight of the nation's health on their shoulders, and very often there is very little gratitude shown, but still they soldier on doing their best.

What a different world it would be if the patient realized that the disease he is suffering from was his own doing and took responsibility for putting himself right! A little know-

3

ledge and understanding of the workings of the body is all that is necessary, but we must remember that 'prevention is better than cure', and day by day we can do a lot to prevent the various illnesses we experience. In the next chapters, I shall try to give the reader a guideline on how to prevent the colds, coughs and flu that are such a menace and cause such a loss of manpower throughout the year.

1

What is Health?

Man is a very mysterious being, wonderfully blended of three lives – the vegetable, the animal and the spiritual, according to the common division of man into body, soul and spirit. It is of course, the spirit that justifies the name 'human', and gives this small feeble body in virtue of his spiritual powers an undisputed lordship over the whole of creation.

Life is a never-ending process of change, the result of two opposite forces of destruction and repair. As fast as the body is built up, it is thrown down again. From birth to 25 we construct the body in which we have to live for the next seventy years, and all our comfort depends on how we do it. The stages of the building are marked in blocks of seven years. At 7 the boy is a child, at 14 a youth, at 21 a man. This period lasts seven sevens or forty-nine years, and at 70 he becomes an old man. With good care and good luck in infancy and childhood, a healthy man at 21 should look forward to at least fifty years of good sound health, when he is not sick and should have no occasion to worry about his body or medicine.

I hope that a careful study of this book will enable many to enjoy this happy state of things, and hopefully put a stop to carelessness or wilful neglect, and by timely warnings point out the disastrous results that follow this sort of behaviour.

If we look at health and compare it to finance, we may get a clearer idea of the great responsibility we have towards this life we possess. The common health is the common wealth, and while for everybody health is wealth, for the poor it is the only riches they possess. No child plays with money so foolishly as many play with their health. In the finance of health we must understand what constitutes capital, income and expenditure, and get some idea of the cost of living.

Capital is the reserve force that constitutes sound health. A

5

person who is dependent from hour to hour on the food he eats, and would collapse without it, can hardly be said to be healthy. The real time for accumulating capital is in childhood and youth, but it can also be slowly stored up in adult life. A person who dies prematurely leaves a lot of capital which is wholly wasted, unless, of course, various organs are donated to help the needy 'bank account' of others.

The 'bank' I mention, is divided into several departments, each of which are so distinct and independent of each other that if we are bankrupt in one we cannot borrow from another to make up the deficiency. In the body, we call them the nervous, muscular, digestive, circulatory, lymphatic, secretory, respiratory and reproductive systems. If a man has spent all his digestive force, he cannot make it up from another system. If his nerve capital has run out, it is no comfort to know that his muscles are strong, and the bankruptcy of a worn out heart cannot be averted because the secretory system is solvent. The bankruptcy of a single system may mean the death of the man. There are thousands of people carrying on a hand-to-mouth existence with no health capital. These do well enough in quiet times, but any sudden drain on their resources by disease will have a fatal outcome.

In health, as in wealth, there are three classes of people – the extravagant who live beyond their income, the careful who do not exceed it, and the misers who hoard it.

The spendthrifts who exceed their income are forever using up their capital, and death will be the result. Those who live up to their income are the wise and happy and are in perfect health, while those who hoard it up soon find that unspent income leads to ill health, not through starvation but through overeating, weight gain and plethora.

If we spend daily on mental and physical force, without strain, producing a healthy fatigue that disappears with sleep, if we are not losing weight or nervous stamina, we may believe that we are spending our income and not our capital.

An individual who finds health bankruptcy impending

usually tries to avoid ruin by using stimulants of various sorts. If it is the nerves he takes strong tonics; if the heart digitalis; if the digestion, patent foods; if it is the muscular system he has massage and exercise. If the bankruptcy is only partial, it means ill health; if complete it means death. Without being obsessive, you should keep a watchful eye on health expenditure, and all runs on the bank of health should be checked as soon as possible. While on the one hand, it is very selfish to be always anxious in every detail to avoid spending this income, nothing can be more careless than to live beyond our health means or to lose a useful life when there is plenty of money in the bank in other departments, simply through one vital system becoming bankrupt.

I have already said that youth is the only time when life force or health capital can be really accumulated, and nothing is more appalling than to see a young person leading a fast life and destroying his vitality through drink and sensuality. An innocent childhood and a pure youth are the best foundations for a healthy and happy life. We get no holiday from our bodies all our lives, but are constantly working on their behalf. They really are a great nuisance, with their continual requirements of washing, dressing and undressing, feeding and looking after in a thousand ways. Happy is the man who doesn't have to add to this catalogue the bearing of its pains and aches, weakness and weariness and disease.

A perfect human being is one free from all disease, where there is complete harmony between the body, soul and spirit. Man is not an erect being for nothing. He is kept erect by his immortal spirit. The material body left to itself falls flat on the earth; it is the vital and spiritual that lifts it up and gives man that lofty attitude that distinguishes him from all other living creatures as the master of them all.

Body, Soul and Spirit

If the question be asked 'Are we body, soul or spirit?', we can only reply 'We are spirits dwelling in animal bodies'. From one point of view, the soul uses the body as its servant; while the spirit in its turn uses both soul and body for its requirements. In animals, however, I think we may say that the soul is the servant of the body; and some men seem to live entirely on an animal plane. While on this subject, we note that while the sensual man uses his brain to serve his body, the spiritual man uses his body to serve his brain.

We have not only three natures – body, soul and spirit – but we have corresponding closely to them three healths, three diseases and three modes of treatment of those diseases. Of course, only one of the three being material and visible – the body – we naturally think most of it; and so long as we are well-proportioned and athletic we think there can be no doubt we are healthy; whereas we may in truth be very sick in spirit. It is a startling thought how different would be the diagnosis in many a consulting room if the whole man were visible and not merely his body – the outer case.

A lot of our present practice in medicine resembles that of a watch-maker who, if asked to repair a watch, examined and repaired nothing but the case, not caring anything for the soul-like works and the spirit-like force of the mainspring within. I should like the reader to understand that the two higher natures of man are as often diseased as the lower and that any physician who ignores the invisible and does not consider soul and spirit cannot consider himself a true physician. Physical health we all understand, but mental health is to most of us an unknown quantity, although it is a special health of the mind that should be closely allied to the health of the body. An active and well-ordered mind should be coupled with a well-controlled and well-employed body.

The health of the spirit is more subtle and delicate than the other two. When man is in tune with his Creator, the spirit is at rest and harmony steps in where discord reigned. When all three natures are healthy man comes into his own and begins to understand the glorious delight of being whole in every part of his being. It is impossible to say where body ends and soul begins and in my opinion there is no physical disease where mind does not play some part in cause and cure, and likewise there is no mental trouble that has not somewhere some physical basis.

There can be no doubt that the less we think about the body, and the more unconsciously it does its work, the better for our health. It is good for us to understand that we are not in charge of this part of the ship of life at all. Here in the various organs of the body are the complicated engines that drive the vessel on its long voyage of 70 years. We can direct our course wisely and well into the desired haven at the end, or we can run our ship upon the rocks at any part of the voyage; but there is one thing we must not do, and that is intrude into the engine room. This department has been closed by our Creator under the authority of a wise engineer, who will manage perfectly well if we only leave him alone. We are not conscious of his presence within, because he lives in the unconscious mind.

Indeed, no-one could possibly be more ignorant of the wonderful processes that go on within our own bodies than their owners. It is a well-known fact that if we want to understand anything about digestion or assimilation, it is quite useless to enquire or look within. We are obliged to go to text books for information about ourselves. We have, of course, the power of feeding or starving this body of ours and when we consider the appalling mixtures that are poured down our unresisting throats as food, is it any wonder that we are not entrusted with more authority?

We should treat the body better than we do, not only for selfish reasons, but for sentimental reasons. It is a good family servant, and has kept the human race going for centuries. It is more patient and enduring. At the same time, it should not be worshipped as a God. It must be kept in its place as the servant of soul and spirit, and those who live just to gratify its appetites and passions are indeed degraded to the animal level.

*　　　　*　　　　*

The condition of the spirit has great bearing on the body's health; we must remember that health, wholeness and holiness are one. I should very much like to leave the reader with this thought.

2

What Causes Illness?

As I have already said, health is wealth, and disease is ill health. There are two classes of people in relation to wealth; those who are content with their own wealth, and those who are always wanting that of other people. These latter lead the most miserable lives and feel they are poor with the same income that is wealth to hundreds. Now if we apply all this to health we begin to see what a large and important subject we are dealing with. Health varies in amount as much as wealth, and there are plenty who say they are in perfect health on so slender a 'capital' that to others it appears very far removed from it.

In running my arthritis clinic day by day, I come into contact with so many varieties of health; there are those who are all skin and bone with absolutely no physique to speak of, and some of these are quite happy, and will declare that they are in perfect health. Only the person who uses the word knows what he means by it, and no-one but myself knows when I am well, or what I mean when I call myself healthy. Sometimes we hear the phrase 'well in myself' – 'Oh yes! I've broken my leg and ricked my back, I've got a nasty hacking cough, but, thank God, I'm quite well in myself.' Of course we know really in a hazy sort of way what this person means – that the physical conditions have not yet affected the spirit – but consider how the phrase multiplies the varieties of 'health'.

The idea of a cure-all for every disease is rightly considered quackery, for what is one man's food or medicine is another man's poison. Certain principles are true in themselves and can be used and applied in varying degrees by those who need them, but to lay down fixed schedules of daily food, daily work, or daily amounts of sleep is foolishness. Those who are

11

privileged to know what the perfect health of a thoroughly sound and strong body means are much to be envied. In such a condition, self-consciousness of the body is almost lost. Every part works so smoothly, silently and harmoniously that life is then a pleasure, and the various functions of the body are also pleasures – food, exercise, sleep. Even as I write these words, however, I think of so many who will never have this experience on earth and whose health income is strictly limited.

Men don't know or care much about their personal health – it is on the shoulders of women that this burden of health really lies. It is the woman that realizes that the children are ill, and it is the woman that can see that her husband is not so well. 'The hand that rocks the cradle rules the world,' is such a true saying. The mother knows that during childhood and during the time of growth it is difficult to have too much sleep, food or exercise. During middle life however, the case is entirely altered. The great pitfalls then are taking too much of these things, which is hardly to be wondered at, considering that licence was the rule of childhood. When the body is built the methods of health preservation change completely. The watchword now is self-restraint, or moderation in all things. When we reach old age, a still stricter economy must be practised. Little food and great warmth are the mottoes for the preservation of health in old age.

There are five simple commandments for the body – pure air, good food, suitable clothing, cleanliness, sufficient exercise and rest. I can hear my reader saying 'I have observed all these – they are nothing but simple common sense.' This is quite true, but our constant ill health is a testimony to how seldom we practise them. The number of man-power days lost through coughs, colds and flu is astronomical. It is easy enough to lose health, but it is very costly to replace it, and loss of health really depends on the amount of our exposure to the injury and on our powers of resistance to it. If six people are exposed to a bad draught in a stuffy room, one may suffer nothing, a second will get catarrh, a third bronchitis, a fourth pneumonia, a fifth rheumatism, a sixth may get internal congestion – six different results from the same cause. What is the reason? It's largely due to their different powers of resistance.

Why Do We Get Ill?

The loss of health is mainly due to one of the following – carelessness, ignorance, and wilful neglect. Carelessness often involves an appalling loss of life, and there are some people who take it as a divine discipline when they suffer, and try to feel resigned, instead of taking the real culprit – themselves – severely to task because of their continued carelessness.

Malnutrition is another outcome of carelessness. People suffering from this are continuously walking a tightrope and their health is very easily lost. Ignorance, carelessness and wilful neglect are especially rife amongst the poor, although since the introduction of the National Health Service people in all walks of life are becoming much more aware of health and nutrition.

Shock is a common and mostly unavoidable cause of loss of health. It often has a disastrous and far-reaching effect on the nervous system, and a very large proportion of nerve troubles originate with some shock. The only thing that can be done if you experience some such upset is to regard it as serious and take rest and change if possible.

Influenza is another aggravating and apparently unpreventable scourge. This, too, must always be taken seriously, for the effects it leaves behind can be more grave than any distress it causes at the time. Its principal ravages are in the nervous system, but at times it seems to unsettle the mind itself, at any rate temporarily. No attempt must be made to resume ordinary work until its lowering and depressing effects have passed, and this may not be for months. The following chapters will be devoted to dealing with this condition and its related side-effects in detail.

Loss of health can also be produced by imaginary causes in a brain disordered by hysteria or hypochondria. A slight cold or cough and these people think they have got cancer of the lung, a little hoarseness and their voice has gone for ever, a slight fullness of the stomach and it must be a tumour. When health is lost from these imaginary causes it is far more difficult to restore than when there is some real disease. One has to fight a perverted mind that is inventing diseases that are not there, and is actually supplying the appropriate symptoms to match these diseases.

'Prevention is better than cure' is a well-known saying, and if disease can be prevented through adopting a well-ordered, pure childhood and youth then indeed we can look forward to a long, happy and healthy voyage to our seventies, and all the way through we can look young and feel young. Physically, young people are supple, slender and smooth, old people are stiff, stout and wrinkled. Mentally, the young are merry, bright and quick, while most old people are grave, dull and slow. Many panaceas have been suggested to prolong youth. Some say the secret of youth is to keep working. Others think a life of ease and leisure is best, but no recipe succeeds for all. In my opinion, a life of faith is the secret of keeping young and happiness is the best tonic. We must add to these two adequate food, plenty of fresh air and exercise.

If we practice this mode of living we can be the proud possessors of healthy minds in healthy bodies, not needing to give much thought to coping with the various diseases that are so prevalent amongst so many today. If you are one of the many who succumb to illness as soon as you are exposed to the slightest draught or dampness, then read on. The following chapters will help you to regain your health and stay in that happy state.

3

You are What You Eat

The difficulty that surrounds diet is not only the general fact that no laws for the average man suit the individual, but that idiosyncrasies and peculiarities and contradictions are nowhere so common, and so impossible to discover in a short interview, as in questons of diet. Fixed diets, except in the case of certain specific diseases, stand condemned, and as a rule do much more harm than good.

We eat more or less a ton of food a year, and the consumption of this food forms a very important part of our lives – to some the most important. We have what is called a palate, and I often think that those few taste buds at the back of the tongue – the real source of all gastronomic pleasure – have a lot to answer for in the way they render us indifferent to what we put into our stomachs. The whole menu of a chef's dinner is based not on digestive requirements, but on claims of the taste buds.

To a large number of people, the stomach becomes either a cross to bear or a God to worship. Gastronomic slaves are sincere and constant in their devotion, and live to eat and drink. Martyrs to indigestion, on the other hand, carry inside them a burden hard to bear. Food has its proper place and the pleasures of a healthy appetite are natural, but care should be taken that these pleasures take up little of our life and occupy few of our thoughts – we should eat to live. On the whole, the feeding of ourselves is not conducted with much wisdom. Our natural habits of eating are characterised by harmful extravagance, a great deficiency of simple good cookery, and a large ignorance as to what foods are of value and what are not.

A large number of people ascribe their good health to the most extraordinary causes. Some say they are well because they have no breakfast, others because they have no lunch and a third group because they have no dinner. There are one mealers, two mealers and three mealers. The 'meal' may mean anything – an apple and a few nuts, some cereal, a plate of porridge, some milk and rusks, an underdone steak and chips or six or eight courses of all sorts of food. All these and many other combinations are spoken of as meals, and people thrive on all of them, which is most surprising. Some say bread is poison – they are allergic to it – others meat, others milk and others salt, while others sing the praises of these foodstuffs.

Amidst this babel of confusion one is apt to think that there are no universal guidelines to adopt, but I believe there are. We began life on milk and then passed on to a mixed diet of three meals a day, and on this regime we throve very well. I think the golden principle in diet is to exclude as few things as possible and never to cut out any completely without first trying less of it. If a doubt arises respecting any article of food, we should ask two questions – first, 'Do you like it?' and secondly, 'Does it like you?', meaning is it free from harm in any way you know of? If the answer to these two questions is yes then continue with it.

We are born with different powers of digestion and the food of some is poison to others. Eggs, for instance, perhaps the most wholesome of all foods, are positive poison at times. With some people the smallest trace of an egg can produce alarming symptoms including a rash and great swellings all over the body. Practice, not theory, is the best guide in questions of food; and that is why so often the patient who practises knows better what suits him than the doctor who theorizes.

When we turn to the question of quantity, we meet with fresh difficulties. One or two things are fairly clear. As a rule, we all eat too much. For years, I have been studying my own health and the health of people around me, and I have found very good health. For many years I have known that a fast is an excellent remedy for achieving good health, but when one has a family to cook for three times a day it is not so easily practised.

The word 'fast' has a somewhat elastic meaning. It may mean abstaining from certain kinds of food, or, as in my own case, it can mean abstaining from all foods and taking water only for five days, after which time I break the fast with a little orange juice. A course of milk food completes the process and the result is magical. Those who have made a study of the fast explain its miracles in the following way. Superfluous nutriment is taken into the system and ferments, so that the body is filled with a greater quantity of poisonous matter than the organs of elimination, such as the liver and the kidneys, can handle. The result is the clogging of those organs and of the blood vessels, and by impairing the blood and lowering the vitality this condition prepares the system for infection – for colds or pneumonia, or any of the fevers.

The total fast may not suit many of my readers but there can be no doubt that chronic food poisoning comes from our habit of overeating. It produces dyspepsia, gout, arthritis, rheumatism, sclerosis of the arteries and many other dreaded diseases. It is quite true that some dig their graves with their teeth. I believe meat is *the* evil in this respect. Fat and starch foods can be stored in our bodies and make us look unattractive. Meat doesn't do this – when in excess it breaks up in the body into poisonous by-products that can make our lives miserable with disease.

How then are we to tell moderation from excess? In adult life, we should always eat rather under than over our appetite. We should keep within the right weight for our height; we should always remember that the less exercise we take, the less food we need, and we should have light meals when tired or worried. If with these safeguards the food is plain and well-cooked with a little animal food, eaten slowly at regular intervals, a person with a good digestion has not much to fear. A fixed time for meals greatly aids digestion, and remember the three rules:—

- Never fill the stomach to repletion
- Eat slowly
- No worry or straining of the mind at meals

How the Digestion Works

Very few people understand the process of digestion, but I feel that I must explain here, with the greatest possible simplicity, so as not to confuse my readers, by what means the various substances we eat and drink become flesh and blood.

It is evident that bread and meat cannot be introduced directly into the body cells without extensive preparation first. The first part of this process is called digestion, but although the word is on everyone's lips, comparatively few have a clear idea of its meaning. And yet one word can make the method and purpose of all the complicated processes absolutely clear, and that word is 'dissolving' – digesting is dissolving.

We must remember, in the first place, that the mouth, to which the food is introduced, forms part of a tube known as the alimentary canal. This canal has three main expansions where the process of digestion is carried on, namely the mouth, the stomach and the duodenum and they are all organs of digestion. Food consists essentially of proteins, fats and carbohydrates and a properly constructed meal will contain all three. The mouth is essentially arranged for the digestion of starch, the stomach digests meats and the duodenum fats.

We will take here an example of a meat sandwich – made up of bread, butter and meat. The bread is digested in the mouth, the meat in the stomach and the fat or butter in the duodenum. I do not say each is wholly digested in these places but I do say that the mouth is specially arranged for the digestion of all starch and flour foods, the stomach for all meats and the duodenum for all fats.

How then is the bread of the sandwich digested in the mouth? While the bread is being pounded and crushed by the

18

teeth, it is at the same time being thoroughly mixed with the saliva. Saliva contains a substance called *ptyalin*, which has no power whatever on the meat or fat, but has the wonderful power of changing starch, which is insoluble, into sugar which is soluble. If you try to stir up a little flour in a cup of tea it remains as it was, but a lump of sugar melts at once. Now the bread is not changed into cane-sugar but into another variety, called grape-sugar, such as abounds in raisins and may be seen encrusted on them. It is only starch food that can be digested in the mouth.

The mouthful of food is then passed on to the stomach. As soon as we smell or taste food the capillaries of the stomach enlarge, and set to work. Very soon a quantity of fresh gastric juice is prepared, and made ready in the stomach for the reception of food. When the supply of food arrives the muscular walls of the stomach start contracting and expanding with a churning sort of motion, and the valve leading out of the stomach – the pylorus – is tightly closed.

The food is thus tossed about and mingled as thoroughly as possible with the gastric juice, especially if the mouth has done its work and the teeth have thoroughly ground up the food; but if the teeth are bad and do not masticate the food they throw very hard work on the stomach and produce indigestion. Supposing the sandwich is well chewed, the gastric juice now gets to work on every part of the meat. By a peculiar action of the *pepsin* in the gastric juice the fibres of the meat are dissolved and liquefied into a fluid that can pass through the living membrane of the alimentary canal. This liquid meat is called peptone, and if you hear the expression 'peptonized food', it simply means food artificially digested by pepsin. Of meats, tripe and lamb are easiest to digest, pork and beef are the hardest.

When all is reduced to a thin fluid mass, the gate-like valves of the lower end of the stomach open, and the partially digested food proceeds to the third great digestive chamber, of which many people have probably not even heard – the duodenum. Our sandwich by this time is somewhat transformed. A good deal of the bread has been changed into sugar, which has already dissolved and passed through the stomach walls into the innumerable hungry blood capillaries that lie waiting on the other side, and been carried off, as all digested food is, to the liver; but part of the bread, still unchanged, has entered the duodenum. The same thing has happened with the meat; part has been made into peptone and absorbed, part has been passed on to the duodenum. And as for the fat, though set free it has followed the bread and meat into this third great receptacle.

The powerful *pancreatic juice* is made by a special gland called the pancreas. This lies just behind the duodenum and secretes the juice at the rate of about half a pint a day. This juice contains three distinct digestives; one for bread, another for meat, and a new digestive for fat; so that nothing can now escape that is digestible at all. These three digestives now finish up the sandwich, and the food is carried off by the lymphatics and capillaries into the blood stream and pumped by the heart all over the body to supply the needs of every living cell.

Food is commonly divided into 'flesh formers' and 'body warmers'. However, a better division is three-fold – proteins for flesh, starch for energy and fats for fuel. I have already said that starches and fats can be stored by the body. In addition to this they are most wholesome foods in the internal economy. A protein is a very complex structure, however. It cannot be stored by the body, and if taken in excess can cause a condition known as protein urea. Three-quarters of a pound of meat protein is the maximum advised in twenty-four hours.

The Foods You Need for Health

All I have said, and much to follow has no interest or value for people in perfect health, who can take care of themselves, and who lead a healthy life without giving much thought to their interiors. But there are some who are not so blessed, either through ill health, or from lack of knowledge who I hope will be helped by my efforts to explain what to eat and how to eat it. I now turn to the food itself. Foodstuffs number six – proteins, fats, starches, minerals, fibre and water, and all foods are compounds of the above.

We will begin with the proteins. First of all, they alone contain nitrogen gas, which is one of the essential factors in every living organism, and without which, as far as we know, no life is possible. Proteins are therefore an essential food for every living organism, and they are to be found in all grains, beans and some vegetables and all animal foods. They alone cannot be stored in the body and all excess proteins are most injurious to the body and to health, as all sorts of semi-poisonous by-products are formed that are the foundation for many chronic diseases. In my opinion, about four ounces of protein is enough daily, and it is best eaten in the middle of the day. Protein food is the most expensive of all in the diet. Vegetable proteins are cheaper but they are harder to digest. Fish and fowl are good sources of protein, but fish does not contain phosphorous in any great quantity.

Bread is the staff of life, and one thick enough to lean on with safety. It is cheaper than milk, meat or eggs, but to derive maximum benefit from our bread we must look to the quality of the flour. Nothing less than 100% wholemeal bread should be eaten – this contains all the nutritious husks of the wheat finely ground. This must not be confused with the brown bread that appears on the shelves, where the flour is often coloured to look brown. The outer husks of the wheat are a valuable commodity where digestion is concerned – they are hard to digest and the exertion necessary to assimilate them strengthens the body and stomach in a remarkable way. The man who lives on nothing but easily digested food, or pre-digested or patent products, very soon reduces his stomach to impotence.

Vegetarians are food faddists on their own. Bearing in

mind that vegetables contain proteins there is no reason why vegetarians should not flourish. However, in the daily running of this Clinic I get a lot of vegetarians who look weak and thoroughly undernourished, and when they give me a run-down on their daily diet, it is no surprise to me that they are suffering from all sorts of undesirable conditions. Obviously, the quality of the vegetables they eat leaves a lot to be desired, but this is not to be wondered at since the vegetables are grown for quantity, not for quality, and with the many pesticides and chemicals sprayed on them they are totally devoid of all nourishment before they reach our tables. The cereal foods are most nourishing particularly muesli, shredded wheat, grape nuts, and of course, there is our excellent standby, Scott's Porridge Oats.

Now, just a little on non-alcoholic beverages. Tea seems to be first in England, but in recent years coffee has become very popular. They are both good nerve stimulants. In later years decaffeinated coffee has become available and I think it is a good thing, especially for those who like coffee but do not wish to take the caffeine. Cocoa is a comforting beverage and contains a nerve stimulant, but it cannot vie with the other two as a beverage, though better as a food.

Water is a very valuable liquid when it is pure – it contains lots of minerals – but unfortunately today we can rarely obtain it in its pure state. Sometimes from a mountain spring or a deep artesian well one tastes the real thing, and one does not easily forget the delicious drink.

This brings me to the subject of alcohol. This in its pure state is twice as strong as spirits, four times as strong as wine and eight times as strong as ale. We all take it, therefore, greatly diluted, if we take it at all. Consumption seems to be decreasing, however, especially amongst the more enlightened. People are beginning to understand for themselves that the corner public house is not the real secret of England's greatness.

Alcohol stands out amongst many poisons because when

taken in excess it successively destroys every organ in the body, especially the stomach, liver and brain, but its evil effects on the human race have not been fully understood. The germ plasm for the succeeding race is so carefully guarded in the parental body that, as a rule, no poison or germ can affect it. Alcohol, however, can and does, and thus leaves terrible legacies to succeeding generations, not confined to love of drink but including many physical defects and disorders. Like all poisons, it has its own well-marked value if properly used in proper doses, but as a beverage the human family would do well to abstain altogether. (In speaking of alcohol, I refer particularly to spirits. Wine is far more beneficial than spirits, and so is beer. Both contain valuable ingredients and taken in moderation are good.)

Tobacco is of course a most deadly poison. It can cause all sorts of undesirable diseases in the body, most of which are very serious. It is very harmful to the lungs and can cause lung cancer. Heart trouble too can be the outcome, because it constricts the arteries, narrowing them and so impeding circulation; this in turn can cause gangrene, and amputation may be the result. A large proportion of the human race devote a great deal of their time and money to smoking cigarettes and tobacco and in the process they are doing their best to destroy themselves.

A Week's Menus for Adults

Day One

Breakfast	Orange juice, an apple and a few grapes
Lunch	Large raw salad, containing lettuce, grated carrots, tomato, watercress, beetroot, wholemeal bread and butter
Evening meal	Steamed fish and two vegetables; raisins

Day Two

Breakfast	An orange, soaked raisins, glass of milk

Lunch	Wholemeal bread and butter, large raw vegetable salad, cheese
Evening meal	Poached egg on spinach, celery; an apple

Day Three

Breakfast	Fruit salad containing apple, orange, peach, few grapes, glass of milk
Lunch	Lettuce, date and banana salad, wholemeal bread and butter
Evening meal	Breast of chicken, or nut cutlets, with onion, marrow or leaks; fruit

Day Four

Breakfast	Fruit juice, and apple and raisins
Lunch	Baked potato, steamed cabbage or cauliflower; an apple
Evening meal	Wholemeal bread and butter, large raw vegetable salad

Day Five

Breakfast	Prunes, an apple, a glass of milk
Lunch	Cottage cheese, raw vegetable salad, wholemeal bread and butter; a few raisins
Evening meal	Steamed carrots, baked potato, cauliflower with grated cheese; baked apple

Day Six

Breakfast	Grapefruit, an apple
Lunch	Large raw vegetable salad, wholemeal bread and butter, cottage cheese; a few raisins
Evening meal	Lamb chop, steamed vegetables; an apple

Day Seven

Breakfast	Glass of milk, an orange, some raisins
Lunch	Large vegetable salad containing beetroot, cabbage, celery, wholemeal bread and butter; fruit

Evening meal   Chicken or nut cutlets, marrow, leeks, carrots; fruit

Always avoid drinking with meals as it has a harmful effect on the digestive organs – it dilutes the gastric juices that digest the food, so that they cannot perform their work efficiently. If you feel extremely thirsty, it may be a sign of a diseased condition and should be investigated. All natural, uncooked foods contain a lot of water and in adopting the above diet you will find that not a lot of drinking is necessary. However, because of the pesticides and chemicals sprayed on fruit and vegetables today – they are grown for quantity, not for quality – we cannot be sure that we get the required amount of vitamins and minerals necessary for good health, so it is advisable to take one good multi-vitamin each day, after a meal.

Constipation should be very carefully avoided. This happens when the muscular structure of the colon and intestines become relaxed, because the diet is deficient in bulk and fibre. The only way to cure this condition is to adopt a diet which provides enough bulk and fibre to exercise those muscles of elimination and help them to work efficiently; the use of purgatives is not recommended. However, the use of an enema should be adopted daily to clean the bowel of loose matter until it can be done by a natural process.

The procedure for giving an enema is as follows. An enema apparatus may be bought at any chemist shop. Put about one pint of warm water – body heat – into a bowl. Then grease the nozzle of the apparatus with a little vaseline and put the other end into the water. Lie on your back on the floor and insert the nozzle into the rectum, then introduce all the water into the rectum gradually by squeezing the bulb. When all the water has entered the nozzle can be removed, and you will find that the water stays in. Retain the water in the bowel for as long as possible – perhaps three or four minutes – then sit on the toilet and allow the water to come out. You will find that you feel a very strong desire to empty the bowels. This method of emptying the bowels is quite harmless and may be practised every morning until a completely natural evacuation of the bowel is achieved, after which time it should be discontinued.

It is most important to clear the bowels daily to avoid constipation, because if this is not done toxic acids accumulate in the body, predisposing it to all sorts of infectious diseases, including coughs, colds and flu, which we are mainly concerned with in this book.

4

How Your Body Fights Illness

The skin, lungs and kidneys are three organs that co-operate and work together to eliminate from the body the various products of combustion, or toxic acids as they are commonly known. Carbonic acid mostly leaves the body by the breath, but some also by the skin; the water leaves the body by the kidneys mostly, a little by the lungs and over a pint a day by the skin. The urea and other poisonous products are eliminated by all three.

The skin

Sponging with water or hard work and perspiration makes the skin act well, but soap and hot water are needed to cleanse the surface. While I am convinced that all over sponging every day with water is good and healthful, I am equally convinced that daily hot baths can be injurious – a hot bath opens up the pores of the skin all over the body and predisposes the body to a chill. In my opinion, a more sensible course of action would be a hot bath once a week and a tepid shower on arising each morning.

Too much washing with soap is not advised, because all ordinary soaps contain alkalis which make the skin hard and dry, and destroy the natural oils of the body. Parts of the body, of course, require to be washed every day with soap and water, but I think a hot bath once a week is sufficient and will keep the skin in good order. Perhaps I should mention here a part of the body that sometimes gets neglected – the scalp. Many people think that the growth of hair is injured by frequent washing – in fact, I think it is improved, providing you don't scrub too hard or dry it too roughly.

Skins of course, vary greatly in their natural cleanliness.

27

Some get dirty sooner than others owing to large pores and loose texture. Others secrete an excessive amount of perspiration, so that the pores get readily blocked and pimples constantly appear. Others again are very dry. Some people are naturally very thin-skinned and prone to sores of all sorts. A fairly free perspiration is good, and it should be remembered that a clean skin is always perspiring and so getting rid of body poisons.

As I have said before, diet is of great importance. All kinds of salt, pickles or greasy foods are bad. The more the diet is composed of milk, fruit and vegetable foods the better. Beer and spirits are bad for the skin, as are pastry and rich dishes.

The lungs

These are a pair of organs situated in the chest, and they perform the most important function of vital activity – respiration. This is the process in which air passes in and out of the lungs to allow the blood to absorb oxygen and to give off carbon dioxide and water. This occurs eighteen times a minute in a healthy adult. We take in air about 25,000 times per day, and this is called *inspiration*. *Expiration* is the breathing out of the carbon dioxide and water given off by the blood. I shall be going into the function of these organs in more detail in Chapter 6.

The kidneys

The kidneys are a pair of glands situated close to the spine in the upper part of the abdomen. Each kidney is about 4 inches (10 cm) long and 2½ inches (6 cm) wide, 1½ inches (4 cm) thick and weighs about 5 ounces (140g). The size varies a great deal with the development of the individual.

The chief function of the kidneys is to separate fluid and certain solids from the blood. It is estimated that in 24 hours the human kidneys filter between 260 and 350 pints (150–200 litres) of blood. Ninety-nine per cent of this liquid is reabsorbed by the body, and waste substances are dissolved in water, passed into the bladder and excreted as urine.

The urine and perspiration are to a great extent interdependent – in hot weather the amount of urine tends to decrease as more fluid is lost in perspiration, whilst the reverse happens in cold weather. If the kidneys are acting vigorously the skin becomes very dry, whilst if there has been much perspiration, as in fevers, the urine is small in amount and very concentrated. The amount of water lost from the body daily by perspiration is, in a healthy body, about half the amount passed in urine, and though the sweat contains little of the waste material present in the urine, the glands of the skin can help to an extent when the kidneys are diseased. The presence in the urine of various substances such as sugar, albumen, and mineral elements shows an abnormal condition of these organs which needs investigating.

In this book, it is not my intention to go into detail about the harmful effects of wrong eating and indiscriminate drinking that causes kidney disease. But I must point out to the reader that a diet consisting of eggs, fish, meat, cheese and other high protein animal foods is very harmful to, and throws a great strain on, the kidneys. If there is also excessive intake of starch foods, sugars and fats, the result can only be a tendency to kidney disease in later years.

Taking drugs for fevers, influenza and such like can seriously damage the kidneys, because they force toxic matter into the system, and kidney disease in the acute form can ensue as a direct result of taking these drugs. It has to be borne in mind that it is the kidneys that are called upon to break down and eliminate waste residues and toxic matters. Very often the task of dealing with antibiotics and other chemical substances proves too difficult for these delicate organs and the result is the breaking down of the kidneys themselves. Taking of indigestion tablets, powders, antacids, headache tablets and painkillers over a number of years has a devastating effect on the kidneys – they all leave chemical substances behind, and encourage chronic kidney disease.

We may deduce from all the foregoing that the best way to lead a healthy life is to adopt the menu on pages 23–4 for adults, drink plenty of water every day, avoid constipation, bath regularly, and get the sleep and exercise necessary for our own particular lifestyle and never take drugs.

I feel it is important here to enlarge on the two topics – sleep and exercise.

Sleep

This is a period of rest for the body, and especially for the nervous system. It restores us all after a hard day's work. But it is more than rest. It is a phase that ensures that the whole body, including the nervous system, can recuperate. It has been shown in animals that the formation of protein is more active during sleep and the same presumably holds in man. It is the brain that controls sleep and the benefit of sleep is most obvious for the brain.

Every twenty-four hours there is a natural rotation of sleeping and waking, and usually sleep comes on during the night when no work can be done. It is not, however, a result of darkness, as is proved by those who have to work in the night and sleep by day, and who speedily adapt themselves to this condition. On the other hand, there are those people that can go to sleep at any time they wish – day or night.

When sleep comes the eyes are closed as a rule, but there are the odd few who sleep with their eyes open. Either way, the sense of sight is quickly lost. Hearing is lost more slowly, and a person can be awakened from deep sleep by a loud noise. In natural sleep touch remains the least affected of the senses, and even the slightest touch will awaken many from a deep sleep. This does not hold good for sleep caused by drugs, many of which have a special effect in dulling general sensation. Willpower is the first faculty to go as we begin to sleep and the last to appear on awakening. Association of ideas and power of reasoning disappear next. The part of the brain which regulates the power of movement is the last to go, and people turn and make lots of other movements without waking.

Other parts of the body as well as the brain rest during sleep. The kidneys secrete less urine, the stomach secretes less gastric juice, the liver secretes less bile, the heart beats less strongly, the blood pressure falls and respiration is slower and shallower than when we are awake. The skin becomes flushed with blood so that it is very necessary to keep well covered up to avoid chills.

The amount of sleep varies from individual to individual as it does at different ages. Young people sleep easily, but as people get older sometimes it becomes more difficult and very often the elderly require little sleep. Now and again sleep can become very disordered. Night terrors can occur in nervous children. The child goes to sleep after a day of excitement or fatigue or perhaps after eating an indigestible meal, and in a short time he awakens with a shock and in a state of terror. The child screams with fear and cannot be pacified. Children who suffer in this way should be guarded from excitement and fatigue and should these terrors persist the child may have to be taken to a psychologist to help him through.

Insomnia or sleeplessness is a condition which is very annoying, and by depriving the person of natural rest it interferes with all daytime activity. It can also be a serious menace to good health. This condition can be due to a variety of causes that act to keep the sufferer awake, or in a lesser degree to produce very disturbed and unrefreshing sleep. People with a nervous temperament can have their sleep interrupted by very trivial causes, perhaps by some external irritation, such as too light a bed covering leading to general coldness, or even just cold feet. Indigestion, due to eating a heavy meal shortly before retiring, or some internal disorder may act in a similar manner, even when there is no severe pain.

Sometimes overstudy, work or grief can cause habitual sleeplessness. The brain in these cases remains fully active, despite the best endeavours of the sleepless person to compose himself for rest. Poisonous materials circulating in the blood can also cause sleeplessness, as in fevers, gout, arthritis, rheumatism and smoking. People who suffer from depression and stress also suffer in this way – they fall asleep on retiring and wake up after an hour or so and stay awake all night.

The treatment of this condition depends on the cause. Sometimes more exercise and care with diet may correct it. In other cases, a hot milky drink before retiring could act as a sedative. For old people perhaps a hot whisky will be effective. If cold feet is the cause warm bedsocks or a covered hot water bottle may be the answer. A comfortable warm bed is wonderfully hypnotic. If the case is studying too hard or worrying over business then perhaps a relaxing game, or some light reading or listening to music may help to calm the nervous system and induce sleep. If excessive smoking and drinking cause sleeplessness they must be stopped.

As I have said before there is a great need for exercise in our daily lives, and without this we cannot hope to remain healthy. The right amount of the right type of exercise results in all parts of the body working at their best. Every organ of the body benefits – the muscles are firm and strong and work at maximum efficiency; the heart works well, pumping blood round the body; the lungs also benefit. The digestive tract, including the liver, functions better because the increased expenditure of energy involved in exercise ensures that the food eaten is used. The nervous system also works well, reflexes become brisker and can respond more promptly to any stress and strain. Usually you gain a great feeling of satisfaction, and when you fall into bed at night a good restful night's sleep will be the result.

Lack of exercise results in many undesirable conditions occurring in the body. These may include obesity, which results in high blood pressure, shortness of breath and a complete slowing down of all body metabolism, amongst many others. In children it can lead to slouching, faulty posture and flabbiness of the muscles. Very often this flabbiness is accompanied by mental lethargy and emotional instability. The appetite is poor and there is a dull look to the skin, and constipation too can be caused by too little exercise.

Too much exercise, of course, should be avoided by adolescents and the aged. A careful medical examination is an essential preliminary to any strenuous exercise. Moderation seems to be the golden rule here, as in all other spheres of life, and each individual should choose the form of exercise best suited to his particular needs.

To sum up then, if we want to keep our bodies healthy we must:-

- Eat the right foods
- Have plenty of fresh air and exercise
- Have enough sleep and relaxation to prevent over-fatigue
- Last but not least – no smoking

Many people now are beginning to realize the hazardous effects of smoking on the body. Tobacco is a most dangerous drug – the smoke has a very undesirable effect on the lungs, sometimes making breathing very difficult and causing a hacking cough, known as smokers' cough. It can also cause blindness in slight degrees, and occasionally proceeds quite suddenly to complete blindness. The cure is the obvious one of discontinuing the use of tobacco. The results are often sensational, and the sight is quickly restored to normal. Tobacco has also got the power to provoke giddiness, and singing in the ears leading to deafness.

A frequent and usually unsuspected cause of sleeplessness is the last cigarette before going to bed. Some people without knowing it have an allergy to tobacco. Although they hope it will help them sleep, in such people smoking irritates the nervous system, especially the nerves of the digestive system, and so prevents sleep. I hope the foregoing will give the reader a good idea of the dangers of smoking.

I hope, that by now, I have given the reader a good understanding of how to maintain his body in good health, but for those who have used up their 'capital', and are forever succumbing to coughs, colds, bronchitis and influenza, I shall endeavour to educate them on how to gain some health capital and maintain a good bank balance health-wise, in the following chapters.

5

How to Cure a Cold

A cold is an infection by a virus of the respiratory tract, which extends from the nose and mouth, via the larynx or voice box, the windpipe or trachea, the bronchi of the lungs, branches of the trachea, and smaller twigs of the bronchi to the lung tissue itself. It is usually accompanied by sneezing, coughing, shivering. Throughout the day and night, air laden with dust and germs is passing over the mucous membrane which lines this system of tubes, and really it is not surprising to find that it is one of the commonest sites of infection.

Tonsils and Adenoids

To counteract the results of constant exposure to airborne germs, the nose and throat are equipped with an elaborate lymphatic system, with its associated lymph glands. We have the adenoids situated at the back of the nose and the tonsils in the throat. Their purpose is to capture and destroy germs settling on the mucous membrane of the nose and throat and this they constantly do without showing any symptoms themselves.

When a large number of germs or an unusually virulent type of germ is captured by these masses of lymphatic tissue, a brisk battle results, accompanied by the symptoms of inflammation – in one word tonsillitis.

Neighbouring glands in the neck may be involved as reinforcements, and they in their turn become inflamed. Eventually the tonsils and glands will overcome the infection, and the inflammation will subside. This may occur without permanent damage to the tonsils, in which case they will live to fight another day. But sometimes the tonsils are so severely damaged by the infection that they cannot adequately resist subsequent infection. In this case, the next invading germ makes its home in the weakened tonsils and we get what is known as chronically septic tonsils, and these are a constant source of infection and ill health.

The description above of the conditions which give rise to acute and chronic infection of the tonsils is equally true of the adenoids, and indeed of tissues throughout the body. Enlargement and disease of the adenoids results in breathing through the mouth, frequent colds, deafness through blocking of the Eustachian tube in the ear, and disease of the middle ear caused by infection passing up that tube. It also causes chronic bronchitis, and sometimes there is loss of appetite, chronic ill health and dulling of the intelligence.

An attach of acute tonsillitis is accompanied by a high temperature and a great feeling of unwellness. The tonsils are large, red and painful and may be covered by a coating of yellow matter. It is not always easy to distinguish between this yellow matter and the membrane seen in diphtheria. During an attack, swallowing solid food will be impossible and the patient must be confined to bed and given plenty of fluid to drink. Gargles of salt and water – 1 dessertspoon to ½ pint (¼ litre) glass of water – are sometimes very helpful. A gargle of cider vinegar and water is most effective – measures as above. I have always found both with my family and myself that a drink of honey and cider vinegar is very good – the honey is an energiser and the cider vinegar a natural antiseptic. Add nearly boiling water to a teaspoon of clear honey in a glass, add to this one dessertspoon of cidar vinegar and sip slowly.

Children today suffer a lot with enlarged tonsils and adenoids, and no one can wonder at this state of affairs, when you remember that the average child is fed on all sorts of junk food, which introduces bacteria into the system and does very little to promote healthy organs. Enlarged tonsils and adenoids are a sure sign that a person is suffering from a very toxic condition affecting these organs, and nothing is going to reverse that condition but a change of dietary habits that will promote health and vitality and will give him that immunity that is necessary to fight off these infections.

The removal of the tonsils and adenoids by surgery is a very big mistake, and does not get rid of the cause of the trouble. It renders the unfortunate patient more liable to more severe infection because now he will have no defence barriers to fight off invaders. What we must all understand is that every organ in the human body has got its own particular job to do, and it is the health of this organ we should be looking to – not its removal. The removing of tonsils and adenoids which has been fashionable in the operating theatres for many years, is a very wrong practice.

When I was nursing and employed in the operating theatre, every Saturday morning was tonsil morning. Then I was trained to think the medical way and knew no other – I thought we were doing a great job, disposing of buckets full of tonsils. Today I could not take part in such an exercise. I now understand the use of every particular organ in the human body and realize that without these organs we cannot function properly, and the removal of any organ – although it may give temporary relief – in the long run will throw extra strain on the other organs of the body, thus giving us inadequate defences to fight with. The removal of tonsils and adenoids will throw open those defences and pave the way for far more serious diseases in after life.

We must not lose sight of the fact that living and working in a stuffy atmosphere, drinking, smoking and overfeeding, too little exercise and lack of sleep, and bad dietary habits all make us prone to illnesses of the respiratory system and should be carefully guarded against. Also it must be noted that drugs and antibiotics have a suppressive and debilitating effect on the body, draining it of many vitamins and minerals, and so hindering natural immunity.

The adenoids are growths of the lymphatic tissue which are found naturally in small amounts, on the back of the upper part of the throat into which the nose opens. They are similar in structure to the tonsils. Very often when a cold develops or there is an acute infection of the upper respiratory tract these growths or adenoids get very swollen, sometimes to such an extent that they fill up this portion of the throat and obstruct the passage of air through the nose and into the Eustachian tubes. Usually as the infection subsides the swellings lessen, and go back to normal, if the cold is treated in the natural way as referred to for tonsillitis previously – the patient should be fasted on fresh fruit juice and water and no drug or antibiotic administered. The reason the adenoids become swollen in the first place is because the patient's health 'capital' is depleted, and infection has set in.

Children are the most afflicted by adenoid infections. The appearance of a child suffering from chronic infection is very characteristic. The mouth is kept constantly open, as the child breathes through it, and as a result the child is very liable to bronchitis. The point of the nose is pinched and the nostrils narrow, since very little air passes through them, and the bridge of the nose is often flattened. The palate is highly arched and the front teeth often prominent. If the child is weak, the obstruction of entrance of air into the chest is apt to produce a 'pigeon chest'. There is also a risk of deafness as the result of inflammation spreading up the Eustachian tube, from the throat to the ear. There is also some interference with the senses of smell and taste. The child is usually listless and cannot concentrate. There is also irritability of the nervous system, because of difficulty of breathing during sleep.

Protecting Children from Illness

As already stated the only successful treatment is to build up the patient's mental and physical health and thereby strengthening his resistance to infection. The following dietary regime for children should be adopted:–

● It is most important that all babies should be breast-fed

from the time they are born and at least for the first four months. If the mother enjoys good health while she is expecting her baby and she stears clear of smoking, alcohol and drugs of any description throughout her pregnancy, then indeed the mother's milk is the best milk for her baby.

I always say that the baby should be fed on demand. I have always found this to be an excellent habit – there is nothing more distressing for a mother than to listen to her baby crying, just because the time hasn't come to feed it. It is most distressing for the baby too, because in the course of crying it takes in an abnormal amount of air and sometimes because of this when feeding time finally arrives, the baby's stomach is full of wind, and this can sometimes result in the entire meal being ejected. If a baby cries, I feel there is always a reason. I never left any of my babies to cry – I always investigated the cause and tried to rectify it.

- Because I had so many children – eight in all – I could not always breast-feed. Looking after the others made me feel very tired and I sometimes felt that the current baby would be better off on cow's milk diluted. This I practised until the baby was old enough to take solid food, at about four to five months.

- Bottle-fed babies should always be given orange juice. This is very important, because these babies will not be receiving the natural immunity that breast-fed babies get from their mother's milk.

- In my opinion the baby should be eating the ordinary family meals at the end of 12 months. A baby should never be forced to eat – its appetite for food should be the determining factor. At one year old the baby becomes a child and starts to walk and take more exercise, so it needs more food. Children vary a lot in their need for food, but I found that introducing fresh fruit juices and various vegetable purees was very desirable. Some they liked, and some they rejected – these I tried later on and sometimes then they were accepted, but I never insisted that they take anything they did not want.

- As the baby begins to acquire teeth, a raw carrot or apple or a crust of wholemeal bread becomes very acceptable.
- It is most important that no sugar be added to this diet.

I have found that, as the child acquires teeth and can chew its food, the following diet worked well;

Breakfast	Milk and a piece of fresh fruit of the child's choice – apple, orange, grapes, etc.
Lunch	Steamed vegetables, or vegetable puree, with a little wholemeal bread and some milk.
Evening meal	Should be light, as morning meal, with varied fruit.

Boredom with food should never be allowed to enter into the day's regime.

When the child arrives at the age of three, I feel that a full dietary regime can be adopted. Breakfasts can consist of fruit and milk – fruit can include apples, stewed prunes, bananas, or any acceptable fruit. Lunches may include vegetable soups, vegetable salads, cottage cheese, baked potatoes, and milk. Evening meals should include a fruit of the child's choice, milk and wholemeal bread and butter, or a Weetabix or Shredded Wheat.

As a child reaches the age of five and starts school, it is most important that he receives a good nourishing diet, and I found that breakfast in particular needed priority. The child should be awakened in plenty of time to allow for washing, dressing and a leisurely breakfast. A lot of children today are rushed out to school in the morning – sometimes without any food or drink and I feel that this is very wrong. Food and drink are taken to produce heat and energy, and in my opinion, if a child does not have a good breakfast, he cannot give of his best. He will feel cold, lethargic and unable to absorb what he should be learning. When mid-day arrives for the school child, he will either have his lunch-box or school dinners – my children always took a lunch box, because by doing that I knew what they were getting. School dinners leave a lot to be desired. From what I know of them – sausages and chips – burgers and chips – they are not to be recommended.

Sleep, of course, is very important for the growing child, and I always had bedtime fixed according to their age, to give plenty of time for rest, and an early morning call to give time for washing, dressing and breakfast. My children always had a full breakfast – fruit juice if they wanted it, porridge, Weetabix or Shredded Wheat, beans on wholemeal toast, poached or boiled eggs with wholemeal toast or bread and butter. Fruit was always available.

In the luncheon box there was a variety according to the child's desires – wholemeal sandwiches made up of a little chicken, cottage cheese, perhaps a little cold lamb and a piece of fruit. In those days the children were given a small bottle of milk to drink at school.

The evening meal usually began with a variety of vegetable soup, or perhaps chicken and vegetable soup, or sometimes stewed neck of lamb made into a nourishing soup. Very often to follow this a salad of lettuce, watercress, tomatoes, celery, a little cheese, and a baked potato. I always placed emphasis on quality and nourishment rather than bulk. Puddings were few and far between, perhaps on a Sunday, but as I said before, fruit was always available – all sorts of fruit. This sort of diet lasted throughout their school years and indeed until they left home to care for themselves.

The regime paid off – my children were happy, healthy, well-built and very intelligent. They all excelled at school, most achieving degree standard, either at college or university, and to this day they excel at their various professions. I feel very proud of their achievements, but I also feel that a lot is due to the way they were treated in their formative years, and for this I must give myself a pat on the back!

As I said earlier in this book, 'the hand that rocks the cradle rules the world', and there is a tremendous responsibility on mothers, as the health of their children is the health of the nation – and as 'the nation's health is the nation's wealth', what a responsible job the mother has got!

The Golden Rules for Your Child's Diet

★ Always remember that drinking with meals is not good. The fluid dilutes the gastric juices and impairs their effect on the food, so digestion is incomplete.
★ Never use white sugar. It should always be replaced with honey or demerara or dark muscavado sugar.
★ Sweets and confectionary of all kinds should never be given.
★ Eating between meals should not be allowed, as this throws extra strain on the stomach and renders the child obese.
★ Milk should not be boiled, as boiling destroys a lot of the valuable vitamins it contains. It should just be warmed through.
★ Always make your own cakes, scones, etc. By doing that you know what they contain and that you are giving your child the best possible food.

By keeping to this dietary plan, rules and regulations, your child should not succumb to the many viruses that abound and should emerge a healthy, happy, well-balanced person for the future.

How to treat a cold

Sometimes when the lining of the nose is very sensitive, it will give a warning as soon as the invading germ begins to attack it by causing an attack of sneezing, which is simply nature's way of trying to get rid of something which is irritating the nose. If you sneeze in the evening, therefore, a little Olbas oil, or Vick rubbed on the nose and also inhaled may kill the offending germ. If your throat feels a bit sore, gargle with salt and warm water – 2 teaspoons of salt to ½ cup of warm water. Salt is a great antiseptic and is invaluable in such cases. A gargle of cider vinegar is also very useful – 2 teaspoons cider vinegar to ½ cup of water.

The question must then arise whether you should stay in bed, stay in the house or go out as usual. In any infection, the body needs as much strength as possible in order to fight off the infection, and there is no doubt that strength is conserved by rest. If it can be conveniently arranged, a complete day in bed or a day spent at rest in a moderately warm room will be very advantageous in order to prevent the cold from becoming something worse, and in shortening its course. Of course, it is not usually possible for 'grown-ups' to coddle themselves like this, but it is the best way to deal with children and with people whose delicate state of health might make a cold the beginning of severe illness. At any rate, if the day's work at the office or in the house has to be faced, cut out the extras in the way of evening engagements and go to bed early.

Precautions against spread of infection

Take what precautions you can to prevent the spread of your cold to other people, who may not get off so lightly if they catch it from you. The gargling and inhalations should be used throughout the day, but medicines for colds which act by increasing perspiration should not be taken when you have to go out into the cold air. A hot bath before you get into bed will induce perspiration, and it may be followed by a hot drink, such as a little whisky and lemon in hot water, hot lemonade or hot blackcurrant tea. Take 2 grams of vitamin C daily.

So much unnecessary ill health is caused by colds that it is everyone's duty to help as far as possible to prevent the spread of them. Children should be taught at home and at school to cover their mouths when they cough and their noses when they sneeze, instead of coughing in their neighbour's face. Coughing and sneezing are reflex actions by which the body makes an attempt to rid itself of something which is irritating it, and if the air surrounding a person who is coughing or sneezing were to be examined microscopically, it would be found to contain shreds of mucus membrane and drops of mucus, which are full of germs. These germs may be coughed at some person whose bodily resistance is so lowered that instead of a simple cold, a severe attack of pneumonia may result.

Grown-ups should not need to be reminded to keep their colds to themselves, so we may hope that people will develop a keener sense of duty with regard to spreading germs of colds and influenza, and will keep out of crowds, and places of entertainment when they are in an infectious state. Instead of saying 'I've got a cold and sore throat and feel miserable, I think I'll go to the pictures and cheer myself up', as so many people do, it should be a duty to say 'I mustn't let this cold spread round the family and make you all miserable, so I'll take my paper and go to bed out of the way.'

Many people have their pet ways of warding off colds, when they have been with a person who has a cold, or of disinfecting their rooms when someone with a cold has been in them. These preventative methods, such as vaporizers and disinfectants are very good if used sensibly, but they must not become such an obsession that life becomes one long process of dodging imaginary danger, and the mind concentrates on disease instead of on healthy pursuits. Fear lowers resistance to disease, and the person who is forever worried about infection is asking for trouble. So don't spend the winter months drenched in eucalyptus, and greet your visitor with disinfectant odours when your door opens, just in case you catch a cold. Keep these extra precautions for times when epidemics are about, then they will be fresh weapons to give you and your family confidence, which is half the battle in avoiding infections.

There are many good disinfectants which can be used for spraying rooms, soaking infected handkerchiefs and linen before they go into the general wash, swabbing the mouth-piece of the telephone and taking other precautionary measures. These domestic disinfectants are usually obtain-able at the grocers as well as the chemists. In large shops, places of entertainment and restaurants, it is usual for this kind of spraying to be carried out from time to time during the day and disinfectants which have been pleasantly perfumed, for example with verbena, are often used. The same procedures may be carried out in the home. Some people like to burn a disinfectant in a vaporizer so that the fumes penetrate through the rooms. Suitable disinfectants are usually sold with the appropriate utensil for vaporizing them.

An aromatic balsam, such as Friars' Balsam or oil of eucalyptus, may be vaporized by pouring boiling water over a quantity in a bowl and inhaling the steam. These steam aromatic vapours are very soothing for the tightness of an early cold or for bronchitis. For personal disinfection Friars' Balsam, oil of eucalyptus, Olbas oil or similar substances of a strong smelling, aromatic nature, may be put on a handker-chief to be carried during the day, or on the pillow at night. Usually two or three drops are all that are required.

When a cold shows signs of being heavier than normal, especially in the case of small children, you should see your doctor. The danger symptoms are a temperature of 100°F (38°C) or more, drowsiness, difficult breathing, vomiting, blueness about the lips, headache or pain in the forehead, cough, bad sore throat, chokiness and pain in the back or chest, earache, or a very profuse, yellowish nasal discharge which doesn't show signs of clearing up after a few days.

Remember when children develop colds that most of the common infectious fevers, such as measles, scarlet fever and chicken-pox, begin with the same symptoms as a cold. However, fevers are accompanied by a high temperature, which is not the case with most ordinary colds. If a child shows a dislike of the light, or has a discharge from the eyes as well as the nose, then it is likely that measles or German measles are beginning and it is safe to suspect an infectious fever of some sort if a child who is normally healthy starts a cold with a really high temperature. Other cases will probably give a pointer as to which fever may develop. Scarlet fever is characterized by a bright, red rash and a very severe type of sore throat.

Possible complications of a cold

Be on the safe side as regards these fevers and call the doctor when the temperature is found to have risen. Broncho-pneumonia is a very common cause of death among very young children and nearly always begins as a complication of a cold, influenza or one of the infectious fevers. The child may be heavy, drowsy or bluish looking with a temperature but little cough at first or the cough may be bad from the beginning of the illness.

6

How to Cure Coughs

Coughing is an action by means of which air is driven from the chest and throat in an explosive fashion. The impulse to cough is the result of some irritation of one or other of the branches of the vagus nerve. The vagus, or 'wandering' nerve is an important nerve which gains its name from the way its branches wander to different parts of the body. Among the parts it supplies are the heart, chest, stomach and diaphragm, so you will realize that the desire to cough may arise from irritation in widely separated parts of the body, hence such descriptions as a stomach cough or a nervous cough. The most usual coughs are those that arise from the respiratory system or breathing apparatus, but the digestive system and certain sorts of heart disease have typical coughs. In addition, a cough may be a purely nervous or hysterical symptom.

In sore throats, colds or affections of the throat, the cough is usually hoarse, barking and 'croupy'. If there is ulceration or thickening of the mucous membrane of the throat, the cough may be husky. If the inflammation spreads further down the respiratory tract to cause bronchitis the cough is at first short, dry and painful, but as the secretion of mucus is increased, the cough becomes moist. There may be fits of severe coughing, when mucus is brought up, and intervals of freedom. In pneumonia and pleurisy, the patient often has a cough, but he is also seriously ill with other symptoms before the cough develops. In pulmonary tuberculosis a dry, hacking cough is one of the earliest symptoms, and the cough is often more severe in the morning. Happily, however, this is a disease which is little known in Britain today.

Different Types of Cough

Before I outline the best treatment for coughs, it will be helpful to describe the different kinds in more detail.

Bronchitis

Bronchitis means the inflammation of the bronchial tubes, which are the tubes leading from the windpipe and which divide, one going to each lung.

Bronchitis is very common, especially in winter and is caused by a virus infection. The windpipe is usually affected, and sometimes too the smaller air passages at the end of the bronchus. This type of bronchitis often develops following exposure to cold and damp, but it may also arise as the result of inhaling dust or vapours. The condition usually manifests itself in the first place in the form of catarrh, but very soon the fever that accompanies it proclaims the attack to be something more.

A short, dry, painful cough, accompanied by rapid and wheezing breathing marks the onset of the disease. There will also be a feeling of rawness and pain in the throat and behind the breast bone, and tightness throughout the chest. After a few days the cough may become softer, accompanied by a certain amount of mucus. It gradually becomes less distressing, and although this cough may persist for 3–4 weeks, sometimes longer, the majority of sufferers recover completely.

In the very young and the very old acute bronchitis may be regarded as dangerous, and the slightest evidence of bronchitis amongst these categories of people must be taken seriously. It is imperative that a doctor is called and the condition diagnosed correctly, and in all mild cases a natural treatment is to be preferred to a treatment with drugs.

Whooping Cough

This is an infectious disease caused by a specific germ, known as the Bordet and Gengon bacillus. It is most common in

48

childhood and most children are now vaccinated against it. This cough is typical and easily recognized – the child coughs several times in such quick succession that there is not time to draw the breath between them, he becomes blue in the face, the veins of the forehead and scalp stand out, the eyes become prominent, and the tongue is often protruded. At last, when the child appears about to suffocate, the air is suddenly breathed in with a loud whooping noise. This may be followed by a second or series of coughs or whoops before the bout is over. At the end of the bout a quantity of mucus is generally expelled with some violence, and in young children vomiting is usual. Bouts of coughing sometimes occur without expectoration when there are enlarged bronchial glands.

Coughs and Heart Disease

Certain diseases of the heart are accompanied by coughs. Inflammation of the membrane lining the heart – pericarditis – is sometimes accompanied by a hard, painful cough. Aneurism of the aorta, the chief artery of the body, is usually associated with a typical brassy cough, which is easily recognized by anyone who has heard it before. This cough is caused either by direct pressure on the windpipe or by irritation of the nerve which leads to the muscles of the throat. In any condition where the action of the heart is feeble and the circulation through the lungs is carried on imperfectly there may be a troublesome cough.

Stomach Cough

A mild, irritable cough known as a stomach cough is often present, especially in children with any dyspeptic condition. It appears to be due to irritation of the food passage or the back of the throat. Conditions which cause this kind of cough are indigestion, diarrhoea, constipation, worms, decayed teeth, trouble with wax in the ear, enlarged tonsils and adenoids.

What is a Nervous Cough?

It is usual to call any cough for which no reason can be found a 'nervous' cough. Often such a cough is just a bad habit, or it may be the result of emotion such as fear, which dries up the mouth. Some people always cough when they have to read or speak in public. There is no disease to account for these coughs.

Many cases of hysteria are accompanied by a cough, and in one particular type of the disease the cough closely resembles the bark of a dog. In other cases the cough is so severe and continuous that it gives rise to fears as to the state of the hysterical person's lungs. As long as other people pay attention to the cough, the condition is not likely to improve.

Smoker's Cough

The cigarette smoker often develops a 'hawking' catarrhal cough. This is due to irritation of the mucous membrane of the throat and clears up entirely when cigarette smoking has been discontinued.

Croup

This is a term which used to be applied to most bad coughs in children, and also to a certain type of diphtheria, so it was much dreaded. Nowadays, the term croup is not used except in connection with a condition which is also known as spasm of the glottis or child-crowing. It most often occurs in quite young children between the ages of four months and two years, and the children who suffer from it are usually delicate in other ways. It seems to be more common in boys than in girls.

In young children the part of the larynx which contains the vocal cords is so small that the slightest swelling which narrows the opening, or the presence even of a little mucus, causing a blocking of the passage, will give rise during the night to attacks of suffocation which may be very terrifying. Usually during the day the child seems perfectly well, though he may seem as if he has a slight cold. Then he wakes up suddenly at night breathing with intense difficulty. He breathes jerkily and air is drawn in noisily, making a loud whistling sound. There is also a hoarse cough. After a period of time, varying from a few minutes to an hour or more, the spasm ends and the child falls asleep again as though nothing had happened. Such attacks may be repeated night after night, but they gradually disappear as the child grows older.

Although croup is very alarming, it is not fatal, and simple treatment is all that is necessary to stop the attack. The difficult breathing is treated in mild cases by applying a hot compress to the front of the neck, taking care not to burn the skin. The compress should be renewed when it gets cool and kept in position until the spasm has passed. When the attack begins very violently and the child appears to be about to have a convulsion, cold water may be poured over the child's face, or it may be plunged into a warm bath. Between attacks, a croupy child should be kept in a warm room, and its general health should be attended to. Anything like worms, constipation or teething troubles should be dealt with, as one of these conditions may be the cause of the trouble. The child should be kept as quiet as possible, and all excitement, irritation and fatigue should be avoided.

General Treatment

The treatment of a cough naturally depends upon the variety of cough and what is causing it, but there are certain general lines of treatment to be followed. If the cough is due to a relaxed throat or some irritation of the back of the throat, gargles, sprays and throat paints are useful and medicated throat pastilles may be sucked at intervals.

Sometimes when an irritable cough is present only at night, it may be due to enlargement of the uvula, the little flap which hangs down at the back of the throat. This cough usually happens when the patient is lying down in bed, because the position of the head causes a tickle at the back of the throat. This is part of a general relaxed condition of the tissues of the throat, and is best treated by clearing up whatever unhealthy condition is causing the enlargement – probably infected tonsils or adenoids.

As a local measure, an astringent paint of glycerine and tannic acid or a weak solution of iodine swabbed on to the back of the throat may bring relief, but the general health of the patient should always be seen to, and you should apply the rules which are given in previous chapters. Irritable and spasmodic coughs are treated with sedative cough mixtures such as the honey and onion remedy given below.

When the cough is associated with tough tenacious sputum, which makes breathing difficult or causes the patient to cough himself nearly sick in the effort of getting rid of the irritating mucus, then an expectorant cough mixture is required. Coltsfoot tea is excellent for this as it soothes the inflamed tissues. Put one heaped teaspoonful of flowers and leaves of the plant in a cup, pour on hot water and allow to brew for about a minute, then strain and sweeten with a little honey. Drink three or four cups daily.

Another good expectorant is my favourite – honey and onion mixture. Cut up half a large spanish onion finely, and add it to half a jar of clear, dark honey. Allow it to steep overnight, then strain the mixture and take one desertspoonful 3 times daily. The honey gives the patient energy and is soothing and healing to inflamed mucous membranes, while the onion juice is a natural antibiotic. Another good cough mixture is mallow tea. Soak the flowers and stems in cold water overnight, then strain and heat the infusion. Drink three or four cups, warmed, throughout the day. This is excellent for soothing inflamed mucous membranes and is a good expectorant.

If the irritation comes from the larynx then the soothing substances reach it best by way of the nose, and inhalations are of great value. The vapour from Friars' Balsam or menthol crystals in hot water is soothing and loosening for this type of cough.

Sore Throat

The throat consists of the fauces, tonsils, palate, pharynx and larynx (the voicebox), and it extends from the back of the mouth to the upper end of the oesophagus or gullet – the pipe down which the food passes from the throat to the stomach. It is usual to describe the larynx separately, as it lies below the rest of the throat. The part of the throat into which the nose enters is the part which is properly called the pharynx, and the part which lies behind the nose is called the naso-pharynx.

The common symptoms of disease in any of these parts are sore throat and hoarseness. As a general rule, soreness means that the disease is in the pharynx or upper part of the throat, and hoarseness means it has spread down to the larynx. There is sometimes pain in the larynx when speaking or swallowing – this is called laryngitis, to distinguish it from the ordinary sore throat which is pharyngitis. Below the larynx comes the entrance to the oesophagus or gullet, and the trachea or windpipe. The latter sometimes becomes inflamed and is sore and irritable, and this irritation, which is hardly sore throat but rather soreness below the throat, is called tracheitis. This is often accompanied by bronchitis or laryngitis.

There is a good deal of pain associated with a sore throat, and this pain varies with the severity of the infection which causes it. The tissues of the throat are red, and the throat is described as feeling and looking 'raw'. If there is a lot of swelling in the tissues of the throat there may be more chokiness than actual pain. There is often a cough, too.

Before a throat becomes definitely sore, there may be warning signs for twenty-four hours or so. The throat may become dry, with tickling sensations which cause the person to choke or the eyes to water suddenly. This type of throat usually develops into an acute sore throat accompanied by a rise in temperature. Scarlet fever and influenza may start this way. On the other hand, there may be an increase in the mucus poured into the mouth, causing hawking and coughing in an attempt to get rid of it. This type of throat usually becomes swollen with soggy tissues. There may be comparatively little pain in the throat and the person may think that the excessive mucus is coming from the lungs and become very worried about the condition. This relaxed condition of the throat is called catarrhal pharyngitis.

Causes of Sore Throat

Sore throat may be caused by catarrhal pharyngitis, tonsillitis, scarlet fever, diphtheria, influenza, Vincent's angina, quinsy, hospital sore throat, laryngitis and other specific fevers like measles. In addition, the throat may show symptoms if you have more serious constitutional diseases like tuberculosis, syphilis and cancer.

The sore throat in these latter conditions is only part of a long and serious illness, and of course, as I've said before, any sore throat is due to a debilitated condition of the body. If the body is kept in a healthy condition and the throat does happen to get inflamed, the inflammation should be of short duration.

In general, if you have a sore throat accompanied by a rise in temperature, you should see the doctor, to get a proper diagnosis, because so many severe infections start in this way. It is not necessary for the temperature to be very high for the condition to be the beginning of a serious illness and in fact, in cases of diphtheria, which is the most dreaded of throat infections, the temperature is not usually very much raised.

The causes of catarrhal sore throat are numerous – decayed teeth is a common cause, as are infected tonsils, pyorrhoea, adenoids and unhealthy nasal conditions. The last produces a discharge down the back of the nose to the throat, which may cause the nasal passages to be so blocked that the patient has to breathe through his mouth. This subjects the throat to air-borne infections and irritating dust that it's not accustomed to, and so a sore throat results.

People who come from gouty, rheumatic families are often easily susceptible to sore throats, because of inherited acidity of the body, and other persons who are in a debilitated condition of health may get a sore throat whenever they are exposed to cold or damp, or even if they are unduly tired. Anaemic people often suffer from chronic sore throats, and on the other hand people who live too well may have chronic catarrhal throats, due to congestion of the veins in the region of the gullet and throat.

Teachers, preachers and people who use their voices a lot may develop sore throats due to wrong use of their voices. Drinkers, heavy smokers and people who eat a lot of highly spiced foods such as curries, or drink quantities of scalding tea or coffee, are liable to develop catarrh in their throats. Tiny foreign bodies may also be concealed, and lie undetected for some time in the tissues of the throat, and may set up catarrh or inflammation; these foreign bodies may consist of minute fish bones or perhaps a bristle from the toothbrush. So you will see that almost anything can cause a sore throat in different people.

If these throats are neglected they are liable to become chronic, or to recur from time to time when the resistance is low. It is therefore well worth while determining the cause of the sore throat in the first instance. When the attack is due to simple infection such as a cold or influenza the sore throat will only last a few days and the treatment is the same as for the disease which causes it – gargles and inhalations of menthol or Friars' Balsam to relieve the pain. Cider vinegar and water drinks are also helpful – 2 teaspoons cider vinegar in a glass of hot or cold water.

You should fast without solid food until the acute stage passes and your temperature has been normal for 24 hours. After that two or three days on fruit only and then a gradual return to the weekly diet for adults given on pages 23–24, including at least one gram of vitamin C daily, and a daily dosage of zinc. This is very important, as it nourishes the immune system, and helps it to fight off any further infection, and it should be continued until good health returns.

White spots on the nails are a good indication of a zinc deficiency and a zinc supplement should be taken until this condition resolves itself. The pain in the throat is often relieved by a cold compress round the neck. A small towel wrung out in cold water and laid over the throat may be covered with another dry towel and left on while the patient goes to sleep.

Hospital Sore Throat

Hospital sore throat is the name given to an infectious sore throat caused by the presence of some germ. It is given its name because it often runs in epidemic form through the wards of a hospital or institution. It is usually more like tonsillitis than a general pharyngitis, and the seriousness of the infection depends upon the virulence of the germ which is causing it, and also of course, on the degree of health and immunity of the patient. A very dangerous germ called the haemolytic streptococcus is sometimes the cause, and this makes patients become very ill in a few hours, with a high temperature and a condition similar to that of scarlet fever.

Quinsy

This is well-known as a very disagreeable experience for those people who are unfortunate enough to get it. It is in reality an abscess which forms in the tissues of the soft palate round the tonsils, or in the large crypt known as the tonsillar fossa which is found in the upper part of the tonsil. Infection enters this fossa, usually after an acute attack of tonsillitis.

This abscess may become very large, so that the palate becomes swollen and bulging and there is great pain which stabs upward to the ear and downwards towards the neck.

Swallowing becomes very painful, and it may be difficult for the patient to open his mouth for the condition to be investigated. The temperature is high and the patient feels very ill and miserable. About the third or fourth day the abscess fills with pus and like other abscesses, begins to come to a head. Eventually it bursts and then great relief is felt.

With the use of gargles and simple soothing and disinfecting measures the patient quickly recovers from his unpleasant experience. Fasting is the only treatment of any value until the temperature has been normal for 24 hours, then plenty of fruit and fruit juices, 1 gram of vitamin C daily and also a daily dose of zinc, after which the diet for adults should be followed.

Vincent's Angina

This is another disease of the tonsils caused by two special germs, one nod-like and the other spiral form, which are always found together in this particular disease. Opinions differ as to whether they are two different germs or simply different forms of the same germ. The condition they cause in the mouth is similar in appearance to diphtheria. There are foul-smelling, greyish membranes on the tonsils which may turn into ulcers. There may be some fever, and if ulceration takes place the patient may feel very ill. Vincent's angina became well-known during the First World War, when a great many soldiers suffered from it under the name 'trench mouth'. It is easily transferred from person to person through contaminated dishes, etc.

So many of the acute infectious fevers are accompanied by sore throat that you should always check whether they are accompanied by a temperature. The two most important fevers in which the throat condition is a vital part of the disease is diphtheria and scarlet fever. In scarlet fever and tonsillitis the first stages are so much alike that it is difficult to distinguish them at first. They both start more or less suddenly with general constitutional symptoms – headache, malaise and sore throat. Certain differences arise as time goes on and the presence of the typical rash makes the diagnosis of scarlet fever certain. In scarlet fever the patient becomes more seriously ill in a shorter time and often vomits. The rash of scarlet fever comes out as early as the second day of the infection and a day later the tongue shows a typical strawberry colouring. The sore throat of diphtheria has characteristic greyish patches on the tonsils or uvula.

Laryngitis

The larynx, or voicebox, is situated below the throat at the level of the Adam's apple. The Adam's apple is in fact a prominent part of the larynx. When the larynx is involved in any disease there is usually hoarseness and pain, which is felt deep down in the throat. The usual cause of laryngitis or inflammation of the larynx is infection from a cold or influenza. Nasal conditions, such as nasal sinusitis, are apt to cause laryngitis because the infected discharge from the nose passes down the back of the nose into the throat below the tonsils and above the larynx. The treatment of laryngitis is precisely the same as that for any simple infection such as inluenza.

Chronic, or long-term, laryngitis is usually caused by over-use or bad production of the voice, and happens most often in singers, teachers, clergymen, actors and members of other professions in which the voice is used a great deal. The first essential in treating chronic laryngitis is to rest the voice, and in very bad cases it may be necessary to keep absolute silence for a time.

Hoarseness is often a symptom of laryngitis, and the voice returns when the cold or other infection which caused the laryngitis is cured. Whole or partial loss of voice may also result from any of the conditions which cause sore throat of the laryngeal type, but it can sometimes occur when there is no throat inflammation present. It may then be due to hysteria, over-use of the voice, catarrh, or general weakness, as in anaemia. In these cases, the loss of voice is said to be 'functional', by which is meant that it is not due to any actual disease of the larynx, but to some nervous or other fault which impairs the functioning or working of the larynx.

If a person loses his voice or is hoarse for more than a month the larynx should always be examined by a throat specialist. It may only be some simple chronic laryngitis, but on the other hand it may be a symptom of much more serious trouble, for the larynx is sometimes the seat of tuberculosis or cancer, which can only be treated successfully at an early stage of the disease.

7

How to Cure Flu

Influenza, commonly known as flu, is apt to be blamed for most slight winter ailments these days, and often people say they have influenza when they really have a cold in the head or tonsillitis or rheumatism, or some similar complaint, so the fact is apt to be overlooked that true influenza is really a highly infectious fever which tends to run in epidemics.

An epidemic is an outbreak of an infectious disease in a community, and influenza epidemics have been known for centuries. From time to time an infectious illness seems to get the whole world in its grips – a 'pandemic' as it is then called – and often these have assumed historical importance because of the number of people who were wiped out in a short time. These severe epidemics do not, fortunately for the world, occur very often, and the last one happened in 1918–19, when the mortality rate in England and Wales was 4,774 per million of the population, and as many as six million people died in India alone.

When an epidemic breaks out, several factors help to keep it within bounds. The problem is a complicated one, as climate, overcrowding, the vitality of the population, the degree of infecton, isolating infected patients, tracking down and eliminating infected food and water supplies, all help to modify in one way or another the extent of the epidemic.

The effects of the disease on the health of an individual depend upon the nature of the infecting agent and the health of the infected person. As far as the infecting germ is concerned, the numbers which enter the body and the way it enters are determining factors. As far as the infected person is concerned, their physical and mental well-being, age and social circumstances all make a difference.

Once germs have entered the body they multiply rapidly,

and give out chemical poisons that manifest themselves usually in fever, headache, rapid pulse, and feeling of illness, which are the characteristic symptoms of most infections. If the germs settle chiefly in the brain, symptoms such as convulsions and loss of consciousness occur; if they settle mainly in the lungs then the patient will cough and perhaps breathe with difficulty. All infections are characterized by certain general effects due to the action of the multiplication of the poisons in the part of the body they invade. When the general health is below par the body is liable to succumb to all sorts of infection.

When germs invade the body and succeed in producing disease the body responds with fever. This means a change in metabolism, and a higher than normal temperature. Extreme temperatures of over 103°F (39.5°C) are most uncomfortable and attempts should be made to lower them by sponging the body with tepid water and by reducing the bed clothes to a minimum. Sometimes in these conditions there is a wastage of body tissue, and loss of protein in particular. The disease can interfere with the assimilation of foodstuffs from the intestine and cause diminished activity of the kidneys, with an increase in the heart-beat and in breathing. Although the skin is hot and flushed the secretion of sweat is minimal. There may be an increased loss of water by way of the breath, but not enough to compensate for the increased production of heat.

Many fevers start with a severe shivering attack in which the skin feels cold and looks like goose flesh. This is due to the contraction of the blood vessels, and of the smooth muscle under the skin. This contraction prevents loss of heat, whilst the action of the muscles in shivering leads to heat production. This shivering attack, or rigor, as it is called, is a method the body has of going into battle.

When the disease has run its course, the temperature falls either gradually or suddenly. The sudden fall in temperature is accompanied by profuse sweating.

When a germ invades the body, the patient does not

necessarily become ill at once. There is a period called the incubation period which varies in length with different fevers. This is the time between the actual infection with the germ and the first manifestations of illness. That is why children who have been exposed to infection are isolated from other children for a certain time. If the period of incubation is, say, three days and a child is exposed to infection early on Monday, it will not be known until late on the Wednesday whether he or she has caught the fever.

The Symptoms of Flu

Flu is the commonest of the great epidemic scourges from which we still suffer, but as yet we are far from knowing how we may protect ourselves from it. A detailed description of its varying symptoms is unnecessary, for unfortunately nearly everyone in this country is familiar with them, either first or second-hand.

The manifestations of flu vary a great deal in different epidemics – sometimes the stomach and digestive apparatus are notably disturbed, sometimes the lungs and other respiratory organs are specially attacked, whilst in yet other epidemics the nervous system stands out as the chief victim. We do not yet know with certainty by what means the virus of influenza spreads. Direct contact is almost surely one way, but it can hardly account for the rapidity with which influenza often travels from one country to another – often in almost opposite quarters of the globe, at a pace far greater than of any method of human travel. It has, however, been proved beyond reasonable doubt that the offending agent is an ultra-microscopic virus.

The only useful advice to prevent you from catching flu is to do everything possible to keep your body's resilience and reactive power at the highest level of efficiency. When influenza is about, anyone who is made aware by a shivering fit, a sore throat, a headache of unusual severity, or suddenly feeling unwell, that he is likely to have caught the disease, will be wise to go straight to bed, and to remain there until he feels well again.

The incubation period of influenza is two or three days and the disease comes on suddenly. In most cases it begins with headache, aching all over and breathing difficulties, usually there is irritation of the nose, the larynx and the pharynx. There may be nose bleeds, and a dry, hacking cough is often a prominent and troublesome symptom. The temperature fluctuates between 101 and 103°F (38.5–39.5°C). The most serious complication is infection of the lungs, and this can have very serious results in elderly people. The very severe form is characterized by the rapid onset of broncho-pneumonia and makes you feel very ill indeed. In serious cases there may also be a toxic effect on the heart, which causes blueness round the lips and mouth. Convalescence following influenza tends to be prolonged because of the weakness and depression it leaves in its trail.

Treatment

For an uncomplicated attack of influenza, the best treatment is rest in bed, warmth, and fasting on fruit juice only. People who nobly carry on their work while suffering from the flu are a menace to their friends. The only way to keep the spread of influenza at bay is to isolate the patient at the start. Experience has shown us that influenza has a trick of becoming dangerous, but with good nursing care, dangerous complications should not arise.

To begin with a complete fast is necessary. The patient should only be given water and fresh orange juice, and this should be carried on until the patient's temperature has been normal for at least 24 hours. Another very good indication that toxins have cleared from the body is a clear tongue. During the fasting period a warm water enema should be given every day – this clears the harmful toxins from the lower bowel even though, because of lack of food, it may show no visible results. When feeding has once more begun, the giving of the enema may be lessened and eventually discontinued as normal bowel action is resumed.

The best way of reducing the temperature during the course of the fever is by sponging with tepid water. A tepid to cold bath is also very good, but the patient should get straight into bed afterwards. I must relate here the case of my daughter, Mary. She had persistent high temperatures accompanied by what looked like double pneumonia. She took antibiotic after antibiotic until eventually she was pronounced incurable by the medical profession.

It was then I turned to the natural cure treatment. On the advice of a renowned naturopath I dispensed with all antibiotics, and when she developed a temperature I applied a cold body pack all over her body. This was done by wringing out a linen sheet in cold water and wrapping it round the body and legs of the patient, who is then covered completely by a warm blanket. It was with fear and trembling I first did this, because I was a State Registered nurse, trained in drugs and antibiotics, and I knew nothing but these. But I had nothing to lose – Mary had been pronounced a hopeless case anyway. Imagine my surprise, relief and joy when the cold pack produced a lowering of the temperature to normal in half an hour.

This gave me tremendous faith in that naturopath, and from then on I carried out his instructions to the letter. The result was a lively, happy, healthy Mary, who excelled at sports. From time to time, I had many serious talks with that man who was so confident of Mary's recovery and right from the start gave me positive hope. Her treatment was a long, slow process, but well worth the effort.

During influenza, when the above treatment is carried out – fasting, daily enemas, body packs to bring the temperature down and no drugs or antibiotics – the patient should emerge in better health than he's been for years, because of the complete elimination from his body of toxins and waste matter.

Compare this regime with taking one antibiotic. Your doctor may prescribe an antibiotic, even though it can't kill the virus. However, it will kill the friendly bacteria in the mucous membrane, which lines the body from mouth to anus, and set up a condition known as thrush. This condition can be very distressing to the patient. It shows itself as mouth or stomach ulcers, gastro-intestinal disturbances and itching of the vagina or the anus, or both. It can take months or in some cases years to clear up.

The undesirable effects of antibiotics can far outweigh the benefits. When influenza is dealt with along natural lines, complications cannot occur. If the reader understands that the influenza virus can only thrive on a body that is full of toxic matter, then it is easy to see that the high temperature, coughing and sneezing are a desperate attempt by the body to get rid of that toxic matter, and in so doing it expels the virus from the body naturally. The antibiotic, on the other hand, will suppress that toxic matter in the body and sooner or later the body will have to make another attempt to get rid of it – only this time the condition will be worse and, if natural treatment is not used, the whole unfortunate saga starts again.

It is the condition of the body we must always think about in influenza, or indeed any disease, because no virus can live in a clean, wholesome body. If the body is clogged up with waste matter, however, every virus and bug there is will thrive in it, and the unfortunate owner will go from one disease to another. Usually an epidemic of flu starts in winter, when vitality is low, but on the foregoing natural treatment the results are usually excellent and better health than before will be the outcome.

When all symptoms have subsided – when the temperature is down and the tongue looks clear – eating may be resumed. Two or three days on fruit only – any fruit in season, except bananas will help to further clear the system and promote normal bowel action – then two days on fruit and milk, and gradually a resumption of normal eating. Lots of green, fresh vegetables and fruit should help to keep the system in good condition. Try to eat as many fresh vegetables in the raw state as you can – cooking ruins the many water-soluble vitamins and minerals. Parsley and broccoli are renowned for helping the body to resist flu – they contain natural sulphur, so eat them when you can. The menus for adults referred to in Chapter 3 is a good diet to follow at all times.

As children suffer in the same way, the same mode of natural treatment should be followed and a similar diet given, though of course the quantities should be smaller. Vitamin C should be taken in supplement form – 500 mg daily for children and 1000 mg for adults.

With influenza, the sick room should be light and airy and should always have an open window. It should never be a gloomy place. Flowers help to keep the atmosphere fresh in the daytime, but are best out of the room at night, as they keep fresher in the dark. To air the room thoroughly, open the window top and bottom; the hot stale air will flow out at the top and fresh air will flow in at the bottom to take its place.

Peace and quiet are the best healers, and those who visit the sick to cheer them up should bear this in mind. Too much stimulating conversation drains the vitality of the sick person, and as a rule he prefers to do without it. When the patient becomes convalescent it is a different matter. He soon lets everyone know that he is bored and his lively visitors are really welcome.

8

How to Keep Children Healthy

An infant requires an immense amount of light and air. Fresh air and sunshine not only invigorate and promote growth of their young bodies but they also check and destroy all germs of disease. Light is a great factor in forming good blood. No infant can thrive, even with every care, in a dull and sunless room, while on the other hand, they do thrive wonderfully when they have plenty of light and air. No infant should be brought up in an airless dull room – the room should have plenty of fresh air day and night and be kept scrupulously clean. Older children should be kept out of doors as much as possible, and well wrapped up in winter.

Rest and exercise are a prime factor in health for all children. During the first few months of its existence a baby cannot sleep too much – eighteen hours out of the twenty-four is not excessive, and it should be laid down to sleep at regular hours. Up to five years of age a sleep in the middle of the day is good. No soothing syrups for sleep should be given, as sleep is a natural process, and any habit formed at this stage in life is very hard to break.

For efficient exercise, the child's clothing should be kept loose and free enough to allow it full and free use of any limb. During the first year infants grow faster than at any other time – they also treble their weight as a general rule. Usually children begin to walk between twelve and eighteen months, and most children begin to talk about the second year.

All parents should be aware of the immense value of intelligent physical, mental and moral training on the character, and it is not too much to say that the future health of the child mainly depends on this. The force of training is far greater than that of heredity, and we must remember that a man is far more like the company he keeps than that from which he may be descended. Two children may be born into this world with equal physical, mental, and moral capacities, but if one is simply neglected and uncared for, and the other carefully trained in all three parts of its being, this latter will usually turn out to be physically taller and straighter than the former, and intellectually and morally there will be no comparison between the two.

Parents have to superintend the building of the human houses of the next generation, and they are given approximately twenty years to do it in. It is true that if they do nothing at all the house will get built somehow, and simply by not hindering the proper design they will do a great deal. However, if they understand the plan of the Creator – the great Architect – and they do their best to carry out his designs to perfection, they will do much more.

The bodily powers – the lungs, heart, etc. – very much depend on the size and shape of the case that contains them, which may be dwarfed and narrowed to produce a faint-hearted, weak-lunged child, or expanded and widened so as to produce a stout-hearted and strong-chested child. We are learning now the value of physical culture for other objects than strength. We find that health, and to a large extent the development of the brain, depend on it. A sound mind is intimately connected with a sound body, and without the latter the former can never find its fullest expression. The spiritual health too, is more or less affected by the bodily condition.

Let us then consider the subject of bringing up children in relation to mental and spiritual as well as bodily health. The only training that can be good and solid must be threefold in character and include the body, mind and spirit. Just as a circle is the most perfect figure in nature, so an all-round training is the only safe one. If you train only the mind or only the body, as some athletes and students do, you create a one-sided personality.

Six Rules for Children

Turning now to the physique of children we should consider their needs under the six laws of health.

1 Cleanliness

A child in good health should have a warm bath followed by a cold shower every morning – this promotes circulation and invigorates the body. If a shower is not available, a warm bath followed by a cold sponging is equally effective, and this should be repeated before bedtime.

For older children sea bathing is very good, provided the child comes out of the water warm. However, timid children should never be forced to go into the sea.

2 Good Food

This is absolutely essential for proper growth. Few people are aware that a growing boy of ten or twelve requires as much food as a labourer doing a long, hard day's work. Height depends to a large extent on birth and heredity, and is closely connected with weight. So children who have sprung from tall and well-developed parents, and who are better fed, less worked and more exercised, will be tall, strong and healthy.

To grow well children should be well fed. They should avoid pastry and rich dishes, but have an abundance of bread, milk, eggs and cereals – rice, barley, oatmeal, etc. As a rule a child should be allowed to eat as much as he wants of plain, nourishing food. When a child refuses food it is very cruel to insist that he clears his plate – he may possibly be sickening for a fever. Again, children sometimes have an aversion for some foods, and if he has to eat them under threat they're sure to disagree with him. Often too a child knows far better what is suited to him than his parent.

Children should not be allowed to go too long without food. If they cannot have a proper lunch at midday, make sure they have a good substantial supper. Three good meals a day is best for children, and they should be taught to eat them slowly and in a relaxed atmosphere. All food should be well chewed and they should have plenty of salads. Pure water is the best drink.

3 Clothing

The clothing of all children should allow the free movement of every limb and full action of the lungs, and good under-clothing is very important, especially in winter. Always remember that two thin layers of clothing are much better than one thick layer for keeping out the cold. Warm woollen socks or stockings are invaluable, and woollen mittens or gloves should be worn in winter, especially by those who have poor circulation. In cold, windy weather the ears should be protected by a woollen hat.

Light-coloured clothes are cooler in summer and warmer in winter than dark ones – dark colours absorb heat from the sun in summer and from the body in winter. Nothing tight should be worn. The true secret of a beautiful body is in a strong spine and well-developed muscles. This gives a poise to the head and an easy carriage to the figure.

Hair should be kept short in both sexes in childhood. This is most important for cleanliness, and in order to avoid the many troublesome conditions that affect childrens' scalps. The hairbrush should be soft so as not to irritate the scalp, but not too soft, and it should be used freely. This is of the greatest importance, not only for keeping the hair in good order but also to keep it shiny; for constant brushing draws down the natural oil that is at the roots into the fibre of the hair and gives it a bright lustre. Long, heavy fringes are bad, especially for the eyes, and they should not be worn.

One word about children's shoes – no child should ever wear an uncomfortable shoe. In the first place, the stocking or sock should be broad and long enough, and the shoe should be broad-toed and long enough. The heels should not be high and you should check carefully that they aren't being worn down on one side only.

4 Eye-sight

Children's eyes should be carefully watched and reading or sewing in a bad light should not be allowed. The proper position for reading is with the back to the light so that it falls full on the page. Near-sightedness is often caused by reading for too long – especially bad print in an imperfect light. It is seldom found in children before their education begins, but may become rapidly developed afterwards. Desks are sometimes badly placed for reading, because the book is far too low. Near-sightedness in children generally causes a squint, which tends to become worse and worse if it's neglected, until the eyesight may go altogether in the bad eye. Any child, therefore, that is suspected of being short-sighted, or that squints, however little, should at once be taken for an eye-test.

5 Hearing

Another matter of great importance with children is their hearing. Children's ears are a constant source of trouble. Parents should beware of neglected head-colds in their children as they may lay the foundation of permanent deafness.

Deafness is occasionally caused by measles or scarlet fever. It can arise from a blow to the ear or from a constant discharge which gradually eats away the ear drum. Children's ears can also be injured by putting peas, pencils and other articles in them, and still more by anybody attempting to get objects out of a child's ear with hair grips or suchlike. If there is any discharge from the ear, a doctor should be consulted at once.

6 Teeth

The teeth are matters of great importance too. A child with

bad breath has a bad digestion, poor appetite and can be in constant pain. Children should be taught from their earliest years to brush their teeth with a soft brush morning and evening, using a little toothpaste. Sweets are great enemies of good teeth.

It is a great mistake to suppose the care of the milk teeth is of no importance. If they are lost too early the jaws contract, so when the permanent teeth arrive they are liable to decay. All teeth should therefore be examined early in all cases so that they may be saved in time.

Good Air, Exercise and Rest

It is impossible to overestimate the value of these for children. On good air depends good blood, and on good blood the good building of the whole body and brain. Exercise increases the chest capacity by expanding its walls while it's still flexible, it strengthens the heart and brain, develops the muscles, circulates the blood briskly, makes the skin secrete freely and is of the highest value to the whole growing body.

In my opinion, the best way to divide the day in early youth is nine hours of sleep, three hours for meals, six for mental and six hours for physical exercise. Indoors children should be allowed to play and romp as much as they like, and they should have as much active outdoor life as possible. The country is wonderful for children – the great evil in towns is not so much the air as the enforced indoor life. Riding increases the growth and circulation, and skipping, rowing, lawn tennis, rounders, hockey, cricket, swimming and golf are all of greatest value. It is good to allow children to make a noise while playing, as shouting and laughter are capital exercises for lungs, however trying they are for bystanders.

Children especially need regular and sufficient sleep – this is an absolute necessity to the growing brain. The bed-time must be regular and early, and to ensure refreshing rest the bedroom should be cool and airy. All active brain-work should be stopped at least half an hour before bedtime. The bed should be comfortably warm and all hot water bottles should be covered with a good thick material to avoid any scalding of the child's delicate skin. Daily habits must be enforced in childhood and are a constant source of health through life. As the child grows, fixed hours for everything are very important, and greatly aid digestion and sleep.

All children should breathe through their noses, as this ensures that the air that reaches the lungs is purified and warmed. The mouth is made for breathing out, and the nose is specially constructed for breathing in. The nose cannot shut out air, and it consists of narrow passages which warm the air before it enters the lungs. It is also lined with projecting hairs that filter the air like a sieve, retaining all the dirt. These kill many germs and filter out others, so that the air breathed through the nose is clean and pure as it enters the lungs. In this way, through warming the air and straining off germs and dirt, it prevents many diseases of throat and lungs.

The mouth, on the other hand, is constructed for the intake of food and drink, and when you breathe through your mouth currents of cold air are admitted directly to the lungs. Because there is no filtering all the germs enter the throat and lungs, and can cause various diseases. Air overladen with dust, smoke or fog is most harmful to the vocal chords, which suffer tremendously if the voice is used a lot in such circumstances. No loud speaking or singing should be practised if the throat is at all sore, or if you have a severe cold in the head, or a chest infection such as bronchitis.

Hoarseness is a very common throat problem. It is caused by the drying out of the vocal chords, from simple over-use which can be accelerated by adverse conditions of air intake that we have just touched upon. If you force yourself to carry on speaking, total loss of voice will probably result and then you'll have to stop – there is no alternative. The wise way is, as soon as the voice gets harsh and rough, to give it a rest at once, and this combined with some soothing inhalation will soon restore it. My recipe for honey and onion cough mixture, given on page 52 is very soothing for sore throats.

Very often school children suffer from what is known as bilious headaches or migraine – headaches associated with nervous vomiting. The cause of these headaches may be some sort of stress at school or at home. A headache, however simple, should never be treated without first ascertaining what has caused it. When the cause is known, you will find that many of the common headaches to which people are subject will disappear with very simple treatment. Always remember that headache tablets are taken for the relief of pain, and are not a cure in themselves – the condition which caused the pain must be treated. It is obvious, for example, that it would be stupid to try and cure a headache due to the wrong spectacles by taking pain-killing drugs. You should avoid taking drugs, as they cure nothing, but very often set up very serious side-effects in the body which cannot be cured. Many of the common drugs have a very depressing effect on the spirits of the patient – they are best avoided.

Migraine may run in families – if a mother is subect to these headaches then it is very likely that her children will also suffer from them. In my opinion the reason for any migraine is too much uric acid in the body. If a mother suffers from this condition then it is quite likely that she will pass it on to her unborn babe, and so history repeats itself. When a person is under stress the body manufactures an excess of acid and this gives rise to these migraine headaches.

Migraines are different from most other headaches, because in most cases they affect one side of the head, though sometimes they occur on both sides. Together with severe pain, there may be vomiting or feelings of nausea, drowsiness and confusion. Sometimes the sight is upset, so that the patient sees flashes of light, and black spots before the eyes. There may be a tingling sensation in one hand, or in the tongue, or down the leg.

Migraine does not as a rule come on suddenly. The person

may have ample warning and normally knows when to expect the headache. The day before an attack there may be vague feelings of uneasiness which show that an attack is coming on. The tinglings and other odd feelings spread slowly for ten or twenty minutes, then the characteristic pain begins in one temple. Sickness, listlessness and so on follow and the pain becomes more intense and may become general over both temples. The attack lasts from one hour to many hours, and the patient generally feels weak and exhausted for the next day or two.

As I have said before, in my opinion the real cause of this most uncomfortable disease is an excess of uric acid in the system brought about by heredity, wrong diet and stress. In running my busy clinic I come into contact with many patients who are victims of this condition. A change of diet to an acid-free one quickly brings relief and very often the condition does not recur. The acid-free diet consists of eliminating the following from the diet:-

1 The citrus fruits – oranges, lemons, grapefruits and their juices – strawberries, raspberries, plums, blackcurrants, etc. The patient should only be allowed to take the following fruits – apples, peaches, pears, bananas, apricots, melons, avocados.
2 Dairy products – butter, cheese, milk and cream. The patient should eat vegetable low cholesterol margarine instead of butter, cottage cheese instead of hard cheeses, and either skimmed or dried milk instead of fresh milk.
3 Beef and pork give rise to a lot of putrefaction in the bowel and create a uric acid condition, so of course these meats are forbidden. Plenty of fish, chicken, turkey, duck, rabbit, lamb's liver and lamb with the fat cut off are allowed.

As one can imagine, with a diet such as this you will miss quite a lot of protein, vitamins and minerals. To replace these products in the body I have formulated a complete package –

called Margaret Hills Formula – which contains highest quality vitamins and minerals, and is free from any additives or colourings. It also includes an excellent quality protein to compensate for any protein shortage. I must say the results are astounding.

Any tendency to constipation should be corrected – not by taking strong laxatives, which can be most injurious to the bowel, but with black molasses. Regulate the dosage to your needs, starting with half a teaspoon daily. A healthy, active outdoor life lessens the liability to attacks, and you should avoid worry and stuffy rooms as much as possible. Women are notoriously more susceptible to attacks about the time of their periods – at these times a lot of women suffer from stress which produces excess acid. At the very onset of the preliminary signs of migraine, it helps if you can lie down, covered up warmly, in a darkened room from which all noise and conversation are excluded.

9

How to Stay Healthy
as You Grow Older

At every stage of life your health may truly be said to be the result of your past life. This is to be borne in mind at every stage, but its truth becomes increasingly apparent as the years pass by, from about 45 years onwards. It is at this period that the seeds sown in childhood, youth and maturity come to fruition, and a wise man stops and takes stock of his physiological position. It is up to him now to make the following years as fruitful as possible; but how is he to do it?

The answer to this question is comprised in the word *moderation*. On the one hand he must not resign himself prematurely to the results of time and loll about in a chair, but on the other hand he can't captain a football team. He cannot do the same things as he did in his youth, particularly on the physical side of life. As far as the intellect is concerned Martin Luther's rule should be the guide, 'If I rest, I rust'. In taking stock of his physical position, he will, if he is honest with himself, probably find a good deal that needs altering, a lot that requires checking and still more that needs uprooting.

It is, for example, a well-known fact that men who have been athletes in their prime have acquired the habit of eating big meals, and that habit continues long after they have given up athletics. With these people their lessened muscular output should lead now to a lessened intake of food. But this very seldom happens at first, and it is only when it is brought home to a man that his obesity and breathlessness on slight exertion are hampering his activities that he realizes something must be done, and that something has got to be a regulation of diet – a very common saying is 'fat people don't make old bones'. If the intake of food is not diminished and the output of exercise inadequate the toxins in the tissues have a slow poisoning effect. The result is rheumatism, arthritis, neuralgia, fibrositis, hardening of the arteries and all the other health problems of middle age.

It is important to bear in mind the common conception of ordinary, more or less healthy living as a state of slow poisoning. It has been said that as soon as a man is born he begins to die. This in a sense is true. He begins to die because he begins to poison himself. At first the poisons which he manufactures in his body are quickly burnt up, but as time goes on the body becomes exhausted and the poisons increase in number and potency until at last they gain the upper hand and death is the result.

How Your Body Gets Rid of Waste

Every physical act, however simple – breathing, walking, writing, thinking – burns up material, and this burning up creates waste products. These waste products must be disposed of, and in healthy people they are. As I have already mentioned a good many of these dangerous waste products are burned up and rendered harmless by the muscles, others undergo a chemical change which makes them easily disposable. The more important of the waste matters are passed on to the main excretory organs for expulsion from the body. These organs are the kidneys, the lungs, the skin and the bowels. However, if there is an excess of waste products the body begins to show signs of wear and tear sooner than it should. It is wise to look for such wear and tear – and have a thorough examination – in your forties of fifties, so that any fault may be found and corrected.

It must be remembered that everything that reaches the tissues is carried there by the blood. Sometimes it has to carry substances that are clearly harmful, and it does its best to rid itself of this material as quickly as possible. However, when the harmful material is supplied in small doses at first and later in gradually increased quantities a tolerance is established, until after some time the blood will accept an amount of a particular poison which, if given in the first instance, it would have made a vigorous attempt to expel.

The blood also helps the body repair wear and tear. The repair material destined for the tissues is taken from the digestive tract and added to the circulating blood which delivers it to the appropriate organs. When any particular organ has utilized its share of this material, waste products are produced which the blood carries away to be made harmless; it is upon the proper performance of this function that the well-being of the individual depends. To go without food is bad, but to be clogged up with refuse is infinitely worse.

The necessity of maintaining the blood in a high degree of cleanliness cannot be over-emphasized. It is very difficult to realize that the tough, solid food which we place in our mouths must be transformed into a fluid resembling milk in appearance and consistency before it can be used by the appropriate organs for the repair of waste. If we try to visualize the amount of energy demanded to convert so much crude solid into this bland fluid, it becomes easy to understand how such complicated machinery can go wrong. One is surprised when watching what most people eat, not that the digestive processes occasionally go on strike, but that they do not give up completely more often than they do. Taking in enough fluid to enable the blood to do its work easily is very important. As we have mentioned before, fluid is normally lost in considerable quantities through all the excretory organs, notably the kidneys which excrete from three or four pints daily, lungs which give off about a pint and the skin, which loses at least a pint in perspiration. This loss should be balanced by an intake of simple fluid such as water, or the fluid present in uncooked fruit and vegetables. Very weak tea and coffee are not objected to, but milk, which is merely a concentrated food in liquid form, has very little value for the work of flushing and dissolving which we are now talking about. Even beer is much better than milk for this purpose. If you don't get enough fluid toxic wastes remain in the body, and build up. The successful cures at health resorts are mainly due to the fasting and large quantities of fluid taken in the course of treatment. Combined with baths and massage these are excellent for the dispersal of waste products.

In the past there has been much discussion as to the proper time for taking fluids – taking it during a meal is said to interfere with digestion. Experience at health resorts has shown that the proper time for drinking fluids in large quantities is an hour before a meal.

The duties with which the kidneys are charged are extremely important. If these organs fail to perform their excretory task, poisons collect in the system and death is the rapid and inevitable outcome. Even when the failure is only partial the results are highly dangerous to life. Their activities are increased when the bowels are constipated and when the skin does not perspire in cold weather they are more active. Nervous influences of various kinds will produce a very large amount of urine and some diseases such as diabetes and certain affections of the kidneys themselves are accompanied by an increased output.

The general functions of the skin, lungs and kidneys have been dealt with in Chapter 4. I feel it will be beneficial here to enlarge upon the part these organs play in middle and later life, because chronic conditions such as arthritis and gout, which arise when they are unhealthy, normally present themselves at this stage.

A condition which I come into contact with too often in the running of my clinic is constipation. Civilized man, it is said, spends one half of his life cultivating constipation and the other half in campaigning against it.

We take into our systems a considerable quantity of material which, though quite harmless, is useless from a point of view of repairing waste and supplying energy. This substance is called vegetable fibre. It cannot be dissolved by the digestive juices, and when it has been stripped of all useful material, it is passed out along the intestines and ultimately discharged from the body. A very large proportion of the matter evacuated from the bowel consists of this material, but a great many other harmful substances are evacuated as well. A lot of these other substances are highly toxic, and they irritate the bowel, and diarrhoea with colic is the result. This is a very unpleasant experience while it lasts, but it soon wears itself out and the sufferer comes to no harm.

There are other harmful toxins which produce a partial paralysis of the bowel and this is a very serious matter. These toxic substances are not evacuated from the body and are re-absorbed into the circulation with the inevitable result that the human soil becomes a breeding ground for any and every microbe that cares to settle there. The result of this state of affairs is the gross impurity of the circulating blood. Every part of the body is dependant upon a pure blood supply and if that blood supply is loaded with toxins, as in chronic constipation, the whole machine works badly and some parts break down. Inaction of the bowel depresses the nervous system and gives rise to a very despondent outlook on life. Once the constipation is cured that condition is changed at once to animation and optimism.

The taking of purgatives is not to be encouraged, it is a bad habit and can be very injurious to the bowel. The only solution is to avoid unsuitable food. The habitually consti-pated person is very often sad. His spirit is sad, and he is sad to look upon – he has got a muddy complexion, which may be spotty, his skin is oily, and his ears congested. The cure for constipation is to eat wisely and not too much; to take plenty of active outdoor exercise and drink plenty of water every day. It must be remembered that the blood vessels which carry the blood to the bowel are subjected to the influence of the poisons they carry, so constipation can become a vicious circle – because the blood is poisoned the body and bowels can't do their work.

The old saying that a man is as old as his arteries is very true, but all is not lost! There is still time in middle age to deal actively with any adverse balance in the body and limit the supply of toxins. The nature of the intake of food is most important and everybody should also bear in mind the necessity for the purity of the air that they breathe. It is in middle age that people begin to dislike the cold, and centrally heated homes, closed windows and stuffy rooms, are very conducive to impure air. These living conditions should be avoided as much as possible, and a fully open window at night should be insisted upon.

Diet

The most difficult lesson for people to learn in middle age is the necessity for restraint in food. In youth eating large meals to keep up muscular activity was a matter of course, and any suggestion of lessening the amount now is regarded with indignation. The idea of keeping up strength should be replaced with the need to keep down weight, and so you should attempt to lessen your intake of food. At present most people eat a tremendous amount of high calorie foods every day. Cakes, scones, buns, jam, bread, biscuits, chocolate and other sweets all overload the digestive system. They contain very little fibre and are completely useless in the repair or maintenance of body tissue. You should also aim to cut down your intake of butcher's meat, especially beef and pork, as these meats produce uric acid in the body and very often the animals are fed various artificial foods in the process of getting them ready for slaughter.

One may ask what foods are suitable at this stage in life. The answer to this question is that priority should be given to fresh fruit and vegetables, together with a limited amount of dairy produce – milk, cream, butter, cheese and eggs – and fish, especially white fish. Game, poultry and any white meats can also be eaten in moderation.

A liberal amount of uncooked vegetables should be included in the diet – you could try carrots, turnips, dandelion leaves, nasturtium leaves, sorrel, thyme, cabbage, horse-radish and cauliflower, and of course the usual salad ingredients – lettuce, watercress, cucumber, tomatoes, spanish onions and spring onions. Potatoes should be cooked and eaten in their skins, as many of their most valuable ingredients lie just within their outer coating. Fresh fruit is excellent and should form a large element of every meal.

It seems that the majority of people today defer the meal of the day until all work is finished, then they can relax and be free from all business calls and worries. Leisure to eat slowly and a mind free from the pressure of engagements constitute the most suitable atmosphere for good appetite, digestion and assimilation. For the majority of middle-aged people a light meal is sufficient. It is a good thing not to overload the stomach, but to rise from the table feeling as if one could eat the whole meal all over again.

A periodic fast is excellent for rejuvenating and adding zest to the whole body, especially for people over forty who are forced to lead sedentary lives. By fasting I mean you should eat nothing, and drink nothing but water for a specific period. A moderate fast might last for perhaps three days.

On the first day you will feel a certain desire for food, but this usually diminishes on the second day. On this day there may be a slight rise in temperature, accompanied by headache and furred tongue. There is no cause for alarm – this is an attempt by the body to get rid of toxins. On the third day this condition passes and the desire for food also passes. An enema should be taken nightly to clear the bowel of any loose matter. On the fourth day you break the fast by taking some orange juice and a little fruit throughout the day. On the fifth day you can resume normal eating. Fasting is a sensible, harmless and inexpensive way of spring-cleaning the body, and it is a very profitable thing to do about once every three months.

Clothing

From middle age onwards there is a tendency to over-coddling. This is a mistake. When you're young plenty of activity keeps the blood circulating and keeps you warm, but when middle age is reached the activity slows down, and veins and arteries fail to contract normally, unless you make a determined effort to take some form of exercise every day. Older people often tend to spend their days in over-heated rooms, wrapped in long-sleeved woollen vests and long legged woollen pants, and double-breasted chest protectors. Wearing too many heavy clothes is not good, and interferes with the function of the skin. This very often lessens resistance to disease, and very often chills, catarrh and bronchitis are the result.

Always remember that two thin layers of clothing are better than one thick, heavy layer. Heavy layers of clothing interfere with muscle contraction and they also restrict circulation. Tight garters and tight sock suspenders lead to general fatigue and irritability and they are often responsible for varicose veins and ulcers. The reader will deduce from all that I have said that coddling and constriction are the two great enemies of fitness and efficiency.

Sight

Failing eyesight usually accompanies middle age, but the disability is quite easily corrected with glasses, prescribed by an ophthalmic surgeon. When glasses are prescribed in this way the doctor can examine the retinal artery. This is the only artery in the body that can be examined under ordinary circumstances, and the condition of that artery can give valuable information about the state of the arteries in the rest of the body. Perfect eyesight is very rare in middle age, and if there is uncorrected strain in one eye any amount of reading becomes a real penance, not only to the affected eye but to the entire nervous system. Vision is the most important attribute of the whole human body, and without the ability to see what a lot of beautiful sensation you would lose!

There is a vast difference between diseases of the eyes and eye-strain – the latter can be corrected with suitable glasses but the former calls for a thorough examination. Mental strain is the root cause of a lot of defective vision, and where there is an abnormality the bodily condition of the sufferer should be carefully examined, together with his past medical history. When there is recurring conjunctivitis, for example, the health of the body as a whole must be looked at. Many conditions can soon be corrected by a thorough cleansing of the system by fasting for four or five days, with daily enemas. You should then change to a wholefood diet with plenty of raw fruits and raw vegetables, and reduce your consumption of red meats and dairy fats. Eat plenty of salads, cut down on the use of salt and pepper and cut out smoking. Smoking is very injurious to the whole body, as it constricts the arteries and thereby impedes circulation – in fact the nicotine poisons the whole system. Outdoor exercise and fresh air are invaluable in such conditions.

Hearing

Deafness is another condition which can appear in middle age, and here again, attention to diet is most important. Ringing in the ears is a very annoying condition. Sometimes it accompanies deafness, but very often it arises independently. Sometimes giddiness accompanies these ringing noises, and very often digestive disturbances are present. There is also a deafness which is the result of continuous loud noises, such as working all day in an atmosphere of loud banging in a factory or such like, and the continual loud noises of city traffic can also cause these disturbances. It is very important to have peace and quiet if you can, preferably in a country atmosphere or by the sea.

Depression and Stress

Mental depression at this age is a common result of an inactive liver and of eating the wrong foods, which produce self-made poisons. A period of fasting for three or four days from time to time, say every three months, brings wonderful results, clearing the body of all those toxins. Cheerful music is very good in depression and light reading is of great value, as are all light sports – golf and bowls, for example. A tranquil atmosphere, an assured income, and the absence of all competition all make an important contribution. Abstaining from alcohol is another factor – it is no use turning to drink to cure your depression, as in the long run it makes matters worse, and once you're addicted it is a habit which is very hard to break.

All hurry and worry and overstrain are not easy to bear now, and the burden should be made gradually lighter, but you shouldn't cut yourself off from all responsibility. Many people who give up work die prematurely through suddenly exchanging an active business life for complete leisure. In conclusion one may say that the greatest causes of the hastening of old age are errors in food and exercise. The errors in food lie generally in excess. Strict moderation in the intake of animal food is important, and you should keep your weight to the average for your height. Exercise in the open air is most essential.

Studies have revealed that women are liable to suffer from stress at this time of life especially if they have a competitive and ambitious personality. They may suffer from stress-related headaches and migraines, and a variety of other diseases such as arthritis, heart disease and sometimes complete nervous breakdown, caused by combining a frustrating work environment with the management of a house, a husband, and perhaps teenage children.

Old Age

I feel that the whole journey of life is divided into three stages, namely the period of ascent, or youth, to twenty-five years; that of level ground, or maturity, up to fifty; and then the period of descent, from fifty to seventy-five years. Old age may set in anywhere along the last stage.

The changes in the body between the ages of fifty and one hundred go on as regularly and as surely as they did from one to twenty-five but more slowly. There is a steady lessening of activity and strength, the bones get lighter and the muscles more feeble and there is a loss of desire for great activity. The circulation becomes less active and the tissues of the body tend to dry out.

A healthy old age depends on three things – structural solidarity, muscular force and nervous energy, and a lean old age is best. As for diet, warm food is very suitable, and wholemeal bread, milk and honey are very good. Fruit should be eaten ripe, and vegetable soup is light and nourishing. All meals should be regular and all excesses avoided. An after-dinner nap is excellent as the years creep on.

Clothing should be both warm and light. Fur is a very good material and wool underclothing is very useful. The feet and hands should be kept warm, and a warm bed is essential – if an electric blanket is used it should be regularly serviced. All rooms in the house should be kept at even temperature.

Old age should in many respects be truly a second childhood. It offers freedom from care and worry, the confiding love, the serene brow, the ready smile, and trustfulness, combined with the wisdom of a lifetime. The experience amassed may be helpfully and earnestly used in wise and loving counsel, and the veteran thus becomes the trusted guide in the house. The intellect is bright and clear, as we often see in very advanced age, and judgement and the calm light of reason shine forth.

The special danger of old age is selfishness – the old man

naturally gets more and more detached from his surroundings and gets absorbed in himself, and as he becomes more isolated he becomes increasingly selfish. He thinks he has done his share for others, and now it is their turn to think of him. This may be true but it is not the way to win love. The aged person should continue to think of and care for others in their little daily wants as well as their greater interests. It will be greatly appreciated, and the love it creates in return will make the giver very happy. He does not need repayment but he will get it, for the pleasure of unselfish love is a reward in itself.

Keeping an active connection with the world around you is most important in prolonging life. Old age has a natural affinity for youth, and having young life around is a wonderful tonic. Many an old person has had an Indian Summer added to his days by the presence and love of the young. If only to attract them it is well worth being lovable, and to be loved one must love.

Old people often lament that they have ceased to be useful, but in this they may be mistaken. No one knows the measure of their own influence, or what lessons may be conveyed by the cheerful acceptance of their lot. However, the serenity and sunshine that illumines the elderly cannot be achieved in a moment. The foundations of a happy old age should be laid in early life.

Caring for the Sick

We should all remember that 'Prevention is better than cure' where ill health is concerned, but where this has not succeeded, we must now turn to the cure, and how best to care for those who are ill. Firstly, we may consider the nature and variety of remedies at our disposal and in my opinion these may be grouped under five headings, as follows:–

Environment

These remedies consist in pure air, light, suitable temperature, general sanitary surrounding, suitable positions (for sitting, or lying in bed). Suitable company, skilled nursing care, appropriate food and drink, and periods of rest are also important. These remedies are perhaps the most important and are really common sense, but the knowledge of them is invaluable.

Removing the Cause of Illness

The treatment here will be as varied as the cause. First of all we should seek as far as possible to prevent further injury. If it was bad air, bad or improper food, these should be replaced by good. If it was sudden change of temperature, this should be corrected. If it was exposure to a germ or poison, further exposure to it must be prevented.

All remedies may be classed either as ordinary or natural, or as extraordinary, or medicinal. With regard to drugs, we must remember that medicines are not foods, that they act on every part of the body, and that it is very easy to do more harm than good with them. If you take them at all they should be given under strict medical supervision. It is foolish to despise them, of course, for rightly used they may have the power to moderate or cure a disease by aiding nature in her efforts to remove the poison or repair the injury – as for instance the use of insulin in diabetes. But if it is at all possible to cure a disease by natural means then the natural method is by far the most desirable.

Treating the Symptoms

It is very wise to aid any symptoms that occure – for instance if it is a cough or expectoration to loosen it and increase it, if it is perspiration increase it, give just a little food if it is loss of appetite. A desire for sleep should be indulged, a thirst should be satisfied, a rash should be encouraged to come out still more. On the other hand, there are many symptoms that are injurious to the body generally; their effects should be checked or moderated. Lives are often saved by bringing down too high a temperature, by controlling violent spasms and relieving unbearable pain.

It is both possible and desirable for those at home to understand in a general way the significance of many symptoms, to know which require special watching, which are dangerous and which are harmless, and then by intelligent co-operation with the doctor, they can greatly assist in the struggle with disease.

Convalescence and Home Nursing

The treatment of convalescence is of the utmost importance for the future welfare of the patient. As a rule it takes place at home, it consists mainly of natural remedies, and its principal requirement is common sense. The regulation of rest and exercise, of environment, climate, scenery and company are very important. The power of suggestion is very strong – it is impossible to exaggerate the harm done to health by not being positive. It is most advisable to substitute nature's methods for medicines, alcoholic stimulants and food in cases of disease. Rest, not forgetting rest to the stomach; warmth; plenty of water to drink and plenty of fresh air should be given full play. You must also allow sufficient time for the organs to recover, and for the nervous system to replenish its energy.

I shall endeavour here to give a few hints on ordinary home sick nursing. In these days of National Health cuts, beds at the hospital are becoming increasingly difficult to obtain and often there is no alternative for the sick patient, but to be nursed at home. I feel it is therefore most important for women to have a good knowledge of what is needed to restore health in the sick person.

In any prolonged case, I would strongly advise you not to trust to memory, but to keep a memorandum book. Head each page with the day of the month, and then each day note down everything of importance. This will include the temperature, morning and evening, the times and quantities of food, the hours for medicine etc. Any peculiarities about the patient should also be noted. For example, you should observe whether the patient is restless or quiet, in pain or not, where the pain is and its character, the expression of the face, the state of the tongue, whether dry or moist, the state of the head, whether it aches, whether the patient suffers from nausea or not, the amount and character of sleep, whether it is calm and refreshing or restless and disturbed. Mark the breathing, whether regular or irregular, slow or quick, quiet or noisy, easy or difficult. In bronchitis and lung diseases, observe the amount and the character of the expectoration.

First of all the room in which the sick person is to be nursed should be the quietest room in the house. It should also be light and cheerful. Flowers, if not strong-scented, bring cheer and are not harmful, although they are best removed at night.

A three-foot bed is by far the best, especially if the person has to be lifted and turned – it is much easier to do if the bed is not too wide. The bed should not face the window, but the light should be behind or at the side of the patient. On the bed should be a waterproof sheet, next a blanket, then a sheet, smoothly stretched out and well tucked in. Two or three pillows should be provided – the patient knows best how to arrange them and they are most comfortable when they support the shoulders well. The bedclothes should always be light – a sheet, a blanket or two, a light quilt, and if necessary an eiderdown. If the patient is ill for a long time, a small light table with very short legs should be provided for meals, and a bed rest.

In the sick room, ventilation is of the very first importance. The air should be kept perfectly fresh and, in chest cases, always at the same temperature. The air in the room must never be allowed to become stale – if it feels stuffy, the windows should be opened wide. The room should be kept clean and tidy, and great care taken that dishes, plates, cups and saucers and bits of food do not accumulate on the table. Knowledge without fuss and sympathy without sentiment are required in the sick room.

When you're nursing someone through convalescence, you should observe the following points. The nurse should be always bright and cheerful and hopeful – but not giddy and given to noisy laughter. She should be quiet in her manner, but decided and firm in all she says and quick and neat in all she does. She should also be gentle in voice and touch, and speak quietly but distinctly, and she should not whisper. She should not rush or rustle round the room. She should not on any account wear creaking shoes – they are most annoying to someone who's ill, and she should be scrupulously clean in her hair, face, hands and nails, and in her dress.

You must take a real interest in your patient, but you mustn't show anxiety, whatever you feel. On this account, near relatives, unless gifted with great self-control, make bad nurses. Your patient should not be worried or fussed with too much attention. Everything you do should be done naturally and quietly. Food should be given at regular intervals, and your patient must not constantly be worried to take a drop of this or a bit of that.

In handling a patient, especially in dressing a wound, the nurse must be very gentle and kind, and never show any disgust or reluctance to do whatever is needed. Any medicines ordered should be given regularly, but the patient should never be woken up to take them. The nurst must be very careful, smart and clean in putting on and taking off any application of poultice or dressing, and most careful to remove at once from the patient and from the room anything soiled or offensive.

All food should be well cooked and nicely presented and any food that the patient objects to should be taken away and something else substituted. Friends and visitors should not be allowed to come at mealtimes, and when they do come they should sit in full view of the patient, so that he can see them without fatigue. The greatest possible pains should be taken to make and keep the patient thoroughly comfortable. However wearisome, unreasonable or exacting the patient may become, you must never lose your temper.

The lower sheet should always be kept perfectly smooth and free from all crumbs because of irritation to the skin. Pressure points on the patient should be constantly looked for and massaged. If the patient is in bed for a long time the skin where the greatest pressure point is, on the back, grows red. It then becomes darker, until it breaks and a deep bedsore is formed. The worst feature of bedsores is that, because they are often painless, their existance is not even suspected by an untrained nurse until they are well-formed. The patient's back should be rubbed night and morning with spirit, to harden the skin. The patient should be kept perfectly clean, his face and hands should be washed as often as needed and a bed bath given daily if possible.

When there is a fever, liquids only should be given – water, fresh fruit juice – graduating to clear chicken broth as the patient gets better. Where there is no fever, plain, freshly cooked and digestible foods may be given. Ripe fruit, free from core, pips and rind, can generally be given, and plenty of liquids are vital to quench the thirst. Ice, of course, is invaluable in fever. If the patient is feeling exhausted, he should be fed patiently and slowly by the nurse, and not too much at a time.

As the patient recovers the return to normal living should be gradual. It is most important that the intake of food be kept nourishing, digestible, regular and good quality multivitamins plus vitamin C and calcium given daily. Regular walks in the fresh air are invaluable, and peaceful surroundings prove very conducive to a happy outlook. In the next chapter, I shall endeavour to explain why it is so important to take a good multivitamin every day.

10

The Value of Vitamins

Everyone is interested in the problems of health and disease, yet there are few subjects about which ignorance is more widespread. The practice of medicine has become a mystery, and this I feel is mostly due to doctors being credited with powers and with knowledge far beyond those which they can justly claim. However, I don't think the members of the medical profession itself think in that sort of way – it is mostly the public who are to blame. They don't want to take responsibility for their own health, so they throw that responsibility on to the doctor's shoulders, and expect them to put right in 24 hours with a drug or antibiotic what they, the public, have spent a lifetime doing wrong, in eating the wrong foods and abusing their health.

Doctors realize that in the pursuit of good health, and in the fight against disease, the individual man and woman must participate consciously and intelligently, but this cannot be done without knowledge, and it is everybody's duty to learn as much as possible about the physical house he lives in – his body. The aim of this book is to help the reader understand his body and to acquaint him with the laws of its harmonious working, to help him preserve harmony within himself and his surrounding. But it must never be forgotten that you are made of body, soul and spirit, and you can't have one healthy if all three are not healthy, as each has a direct bearing on the other.

Our goal in life is to become holy. Holiness means wholeness, and in order to become truly whole we have to keep growing, readjusting and changing, in order to explore and discover all that is within us. Only then can we reach our full potential as children of God. But by middle age, we have become tired. We have probably invested many years, much time and energy and emotion in our work, our family or our faith, and yet we may feel that we have very little to show for it. At work we may not have achieved all we originally hoped for. Our family life may not have turned out as we had expected or planned for and our faith may well have become a habit and a routine which brings us little more than a sense of safety in the hour of death.

In the face of all this it is hardly surprising that midlife brings with it a sense of depression and impending crisis. Crisis, though, can mean a turning point, a time of decision, of change – a time to adjust or readjust to a new reality. We have to be patient with ourselves and with others. The gift of hope can sustain us through the long years of middle age, as we face the changes in ourselves and in others. Gradually we move from being rather closed-in people in terms of life and faith, towards developing an increasing ability to love and let go. In the experience of defeat in many areas of our lives we will begin to experience also a sense of new beginnings, new life and continuous creation, in partnership with God.

The reader may well ask what all this has to do with good health and how to attain it, and having attained it how to keep it. The answer is that, as I have said before, the health of the body has a direct bearing on the health of the soul and spirit.

The reason I associate a spiritual thinking with middle age in particular, is because most of us are too busy building a home and family, trying to excel at work, thinking about success or failure in our careers, to give much thought to who we are. It is usually in middle age that this machine we call our body begins to break down, and we then look back and take stock of how wrongly we have treated this body of ours – wrong food, drink, not enough rest and so on. But all is not lost – we can experience a new beginning, resolve to eat the right foods, take adequate exercise and rest and – very important – teach others to do the same.

In this chapter, I propose to speak mainly of vitamins and their relation to bodily health. The presence of these substances in our food is essential to healthy growth, and the absence of any one of them over a period of time results in a characteristic disease. Rickets, caused by a shortage of vitamin D, and scurvy, due to the absence of vitamin C, are both examples of this.

The need for a balanced diet begins at birth. The presence of the necessary vitamins in breast milk depends upon the mother's diet; if the mother's diet contains a sufficiency of all the vitamins they are secreted in the milk. Thus the milk of a mother who includes in her diet a daily ration of fresh milk, butter, eggs and animal fats, will contain sufficent vitamin D to protect her infant from rickets. The children of poor mothers, who substitute margarine for butter, skimmed milk for whole fresh milk and to whom eggs and meat are rare luxuries, may well grow up with weak bones. There are some diseases in which these fresh dairy products are not permissible, such as gall bladder conditions, arthritis and skin rashes, and in all such cases supplements of vitamin D should be taken.

One vitamin cannot deputize for another. Vitamin A, for instance, cannot replace vitamin B, and if for a prolonged period of time any of these vitamins are not supplied in the food, very serious consequences to health may be the result. It is very important to remember that vitamins are present only in minute quantities in any of the foodstuffs (though more in some than in others) and that they are very easily removed from foods by the milling of grain, soaking in water and cooking – especially for long periods – and some are completely destroyed by certain chemicals.

All vitamins are formed primarily in plants, and the vitamins found in animal tissues are derived from the plants on which these animals have fed. It is clear, therefore, from the vitamin point of view that vegetable foods have a decided advantage over animal foods. Not many of the individual foods contain all the vitamins. Vitamin A, for example, is found in green vegetables and in all the animal fats except lard. Vitamin B is found principally in the seeds of plants, and in the eggs and internal organs of animals. Vitamin C is present in all fresh fruit and vegetables. Vitamin D is nearly always to be found with vitamin A in animal fats. Codliver oil and halibut liver oil are especially rich in vitamins A and D. The best fruits for the supply of vitamin C are oranges, lemons, tomatoes, pineapples, apples and bananas. Grapes are very low in vitamin C. The vegetables which contain this vitamin in greatest abundance are watercress, spinach, cabbage, green peas, cucumber and carrots. Cooking, although it does not in every case destroy vitamins, is very liable to minimize their quality, so of course, it is much better to eat vegetables raw.

The Value of Vitamin C

In the treatment of coughs, colds and flu, vitamin C claims first place. It is vital to keep the immune system healthy and ward off infection. This vitamin is found in citrus fruits, tomatoes, potatoes and leafy green vegetables. It is very easily destroyed in the presence of air and in cooking, especially when bicarbonate of soda is added in the cooking. In man, the daily requirement of vitamin C is supposed to be one mg per kg of bodyweight, and about twice that amount for babies and pregnant women. It is not stored in the body, so you need to take it every day, and a higher intake is desirable during illness, when the body uses more of it.

Doses of 1 g or more per day are reputed to prevent or cure the common cold, and I must agree that I have got the utmost faith in its efficacy. When I feel a cold coming on I reach for the vitamin C at once – and thankfully it never seems to develop. I take 2 g throughout the day until all symptoms have passed and then reduce to 1 g daily. I take this every day, and I can't remember when I last had a cold.

The most extreme result of a deficiency is scurvy, a disease where the body tissues break down. However, a shortage can also cause colds, bronchitis, asthma, indigestion and slow healing of wounds. It can also cause stress, and people who are under stress are advised to take 2 g daily – 500 mg at breakfast, 1000 mg at lunch and 500 mg in the evening – to combat the effects of stress.

Unfortunately, most of us don't eat as many fresh fruits and vegetables as we should, and very few of us eat the skins, membranes and rinds of citrus fruits, which are among the richest sources of vitamin C. Increasing our intake of this important vitamin could clear up a host of nagging health problems. Vitamin C strengthens the capillary walls – the walls of blood vessels – so we may assume from this that people who get persistent nose-bleeds could benefit. It is my belief that some miscarriages occur because of weakening of the capillaries in the placenta, so it stands to reason that any substance that will strengthen and toughen the walls of these capillaries will help in these circumstances.

Vitamin C also plays a very important part in the formation of collagen in the body cells – this is very important for the growth and repair of all cells, and teeth, blood vessels, and bones all benefit from it. It is also very important in helping the absorption of iron in the body – without vitamin C, iron can affect the liver, and cause liver poisoning. Smokers and those who eat white sugar deplete the vitamin C in their bodies, and these groups of people should take more than the recommended daily allowance.

The following are a list of the many uses of vitamin C:-

★ It helps prevent the common cold.
★ It acts as a natural laxative.
★ It prevents scurvy.
★ It helps prevent infections.
★ It helps in the formation of collagen in bodily cells and tissues.
★ It helps to prevent blood clots.
★ It helps in the healing of wounds.

Natural vitamin C is the best form to take, as this is the most easily absorbed by the body, and these are supplied in tablet form, usually in strengths of 500 mg (half a gram). Rosehips are the richest natural source of the vitamin. It is very difficult to take too much vitamin C, but if you do it can have side-effects such as diarrhoea and skin rashes. Women who are on the pill should take extra vitamin C daily. Pain relievers such as aspirin and paracetamol, and most other drugs, destroy this vitamin in the body, so large doses of approx. 2000 mg should be taken daily to counteract this.

Vitamin C is reputed to be invaluable in the prevention and treatment of cancer and it is invaluable for cancer patients who are undergoing chemotherapy and radiation treatment, because they wreck the immune system, and only large doses of vitamin C can help protect it. It is also a good natural anti-histamine – it is invaluable in the treatment of cold sores, influenza and bronchial asthma. In the hay-fever season it wards off attacks and by strengthening the capillary walls it prevents nose bleeds.

Multivitamins

In my opinion, everybody should take a good multivitamin and mineral tablet each day to ensure good health. This should include the following vitamins:

Vitamin A – 200 International Units
Vitamin B1 – 100 milligrams
Vitamin B2 – 100 milligrams
Nicotinamide – 100 milligrams
Vitamin B6 – 100 milligrams
Vitamin D – 2000 International Units
Calcium – 500 milligrams
Vitamin E – 200 International Units

In these days of growing food for quantity instead of quality, when nearly all our fruit and vegetables are being sprayed with pesticides and chemicals, it is no wonder that a host of deficiency diseases, for example cancer and arthritis, amongst a lot of others, are common, because the vitamins and minerals that we should be getting from our food are destroyed before it reaches our tables.

All through our lives our body processes are at the mercy of the food we eat, and a bad balance in the diet may cause serious and cumulative trouble. It is probable that most of us are in little danger of the acute diseases which are caused by deficiency of one or another of the vitamins, but the possibility of troubles due to minor but continued deficiencies are less remote.

Our occupation affects our environment. We spend much of our lives at work, and if our occupation is too arduous for our particular powers, or if our work is in unsuitable conditions, our health must be affected. Excesses of dust, fumes, heat or damp bring their troubles, and lack of air and sunlight are as harmful at work as at home.

Occupation affects our functions – the use or disuse of our parts or qualities. Use or education of an organ or a mental quality leads to its development, while disuse may lead to deterioration – in other words, if you don't want to lose it, use it. We cannot develop anything which our hereditary equipment does not supply. But suitable environment, use and wise guidance can do much to make the best of the available material, to encourage the good qualities and to suppress the less desirable elements. We can certainly do a lot to control our health and our lives.

Vitamins A & D

These vitamins are nearly always found together in animal fats such as suet, dripping, lard, bacon fat, butter, cream, and egg yolk, in vegetable fats such as olive oil, cotton-seed oil, nut butters and margarine, and in fish fats such as codliver oil and halibut oil. Fats are necessary in all diets, but needs vary.

Vitamin A is essential for growth and protects against infection, while vitamin D protects against rickets, and a lack of it may prevent the child's teeth and gums from developing as they should.

Vitamin B

As I have said before, this vitamin is found principally in the seeds of plants, and in the eggs and internal organs of animals. It is a complex vitamin – it is really a combination of nutrients all working together, to produce good health and especially healthy nerves. I feel that it is not necessary to enlarge on the various individual nutrients that go to make up B complex here. I think it is sufficient to say what dangers a lack of it can lead to.

The main symptoms of vitamin B deficiency are sleeplessness, lack of appetitite, indigestion, constipation, swollen ankles, weakness of the heart muscle, diarrhoea, memory disturbance, irritability, eye problems, premature senility, stiffness of the joints and tiredness, diabetes mellitus, asthma and kidney stones, pain and weakness in the hands with numbness and tingling of the fingers, hardening of the arteries, angina, stress, night blindness, osteoporosis, reduction of fertility, migraine headaches and depression.

Vitamin E

This is a most essential vitamin in our daily life. It is mostly renowned for modifying blood fats and so protecting against heart disease, but its use does not stop there. It helps the circulation, and helps the immune system – defending us from coughs, colds, flu and many more serious diseases.

In the running of my busy clinic for arthritics, I come across various symptoms and illnesses. A lot of my patients suffer from very severe cramps, especially at night, in the feet and legs. I give them all 400 International Units daily, and in a very short time they not only get relief from their cramps, but they report a definite lessening of cold in their hands and feet, thereby showing me that their circulation is benefiting as well.

Some of my patients suffer with deep vein thrombosis, others with phlebitis – these are very painful conditions, and in my opinion both are due to deposits of cholesterol which block the flow of blood. I always give 400 International Units of vitamin E in conjunction with lecithin to these patients. The lecithin helps dissolve the cholesterol and the vitamin E increases the circulation, and sometimes I am astounded at the good results obtained.

It is most important that patients who have had a stroke should have these two supplements because a stroke is caused by deposits of cholesterol lodging in the brain and so impeding the blood flow. It stands to reason that something that will disperse these cholesterol deposits and improve circulation makes good sense and should be administered to the patient. Sometimes a clot may lodge in the lungs, causing pulmonary embolism – this too, is a very serious condition, and the same treatment applies.

As you may deduce from all this, vitamin E has many, many uses throughout the body – it helps in migraine headaches, relieves stress, helps cure cold sores, relieves burns and shock, and it helps protect the eyes in patients suffering from diabetes.

Calcium

This is a mineral which is of the utmost importance in the body for building and repairing bones and teeth, for muscle function, especially for the heart muscle, for proper blood clotting and in the transmission of nerve impulses. For people suffering from high histamine levels, it is said to lower the histamine and relieve the constant headaches associated with the condition.

Calcium helps the absorption of vitamin D in the body, and

regulates the amount of bone-building material absorbed through the intestines. When the bones are starved of this bone-building material they become brittle – a condition known as osteoporosis. This is widespread in people over forty years of age, and especially common in post-menopausal women over forty-five. It is a known fact that this category of women often break their hips and thighs, because their bones are so brittle.

Lack of calcium in the body not only interferes with the health of the bones but also makes the skin dry and the nails brittle and ridged; it produces dry, lustreless hair, dry eyes and unhealthy teeth and gums. In my opinion, everybody over 40 years of age should be taking a good calcium supplement. My experience in running my clinic for arthritics has taught me that the vast majority suffer from oesteoporosis and giving them high dosages of natural calcium, combined, of course, with other natural combinations of vitamins, produces an improvement in a very short time, and they go on improving, some to become totally clear of arthritis.

11

Stress and Your Health

I feel it is very important to discuss stress, and the underlying effect it has in coughs, colds and flu, and indeed in all diseases. Stress comes in many forms throughout our lives, from the cradle to the grave, and it seems unavoidable – we all get it in one form or another. In infancy, there are the stress cries sent out by the baby who needs changing or feeding, who is suffering with wind in his tummy that needs getting up, or perhaps he is suffering from too much heat or too much cold. The only way he can attract attention is to keep on crying until something is done to put things right. Then there is the young inexperienced mum under stress because she doesn't know why her baby is crying. As the baby grows there are all the childhood ailments to deal with, plus all the coughs, colds, rashes, high temperatures – all sources of stress for both mother and child.

A lot of us don't realize that as the child starts school a great deal of stress is caused. His mother wonders whether he will mix well, if he can tie his shoe laces properly, if he'll eat his lunch – there are so many things to worry about. The child is very apprehensive about his new surroundings and would much rather be at home with his mum. There are the school dinners – not the same as mum cooks, but he has to eat them, and sometimes a nervousness is set up which produces a cough, a cold or a tummy ache, all because of stress.

Growing up further brings more stress; those exams, the competition, the comparisons within the family – why can't Johnny be as good as his elder brother? Why doesn't he like games? – the criticism from parents and teachers seem never-ending. At home Mum is undergoing her own stress, as she has taken a part-time job, so as well as bringing up Johnny and his brother, she's working in a stuffy office, for very little money. Perhaps she doesn't want to work, and the house-work, washing, cleaning, polishing, ironing and cooking have still got to be fitted in, in the evening when she comes home; but she bravely carries on under tremendous stress, worn out, but trying to prove she's the woman of the year. She feels guilty if everything is not in tip-top order, and if she can't cope she refuses to admit it. Weekends are spent shopping – pandering to the family's whims and trying very hard to be the glamour-girl her husband married.

The amount of stress involved in this sort of living is astronomical, and the body and mind can't take it. Minor symptoms begin to appear – headaches, colds, flu, neck, back and shoulder pains, chronic fatigue, and premenstrual tension. It's time to slow down, but the feelings of inadequacy won't let her do this, so the doctor's surgery is the next step. She complains of headaches, sleepless nights, tiredness, fraught nerves, so she comes out of the surgery with a prescription for Valium or some such drug. Now she really is in trouble – the taking of this drug may lead to dependence on it, and the side-effects it produces can play havoc with her life, and all because she has been driving herself too hard – and the stress has proved too much.

So far we haven't mentioned Johnny's father, a portly businessman who devours expense account lunches and dinners, smokes cigars and sits behind his executive desk working late every day. Of course, his whole system will become lethargic, his heart and blood pressure will be at risk, hardening of the arteries may set in, and the smoking may contribute to lung cancer. However, Johnny's mother may be more liable than her husband to suffer from stress, because she is of a highly competitive and ambitious personality. She must learn to love herself and take loving care of her body.

The essential thing to do is to find some balance in your life, and to find out just how much stress you can take. Everybody differs here – what may be too much stress for one may have no effect whatsoever on another. Positive stress is a good thing – it keeps us from getting bored and promotes energy – but when we overstep this stress level the danger signals set in – headaches and tension appear, and acting and thinking quickly or clearly become impossible.

Relaxation and exercise are a good way to handle the negative effects of stress. Any type of stress alerts the body for action and if no action is taken large amounts of fatty acids build up in the blood stream, very often raising the blood pressure. Anxiety, hostility or any sort of tenseness call for more exercise out in the fresh air if at all possible. Meditation, relaxation and deep breathing also help to minimize stress levels. Try and see the funny side of life, and look on stressful situations as challenges, not as problems that cannot be surmounted.

Turning to coffee, cigarettes or alcohol won't help, and Valium and all other tranquillisers should be avoided – they may ease the symptoms for a while, but the cause will not have been removed. A well-balanced diet is always necessary to maintain good health. Physical and mental stress very often depletes vitamin B complex in the system, thereby depriving the nerves of their food, so 100 mg should be taken daily in supplement form to top up what we get from our food. Calcium too is very necessary, as this is vital for healthy nerves and muscles. Zinc is also very important, as zinc nourishes the immune system and helps it to fight off all those cough, colds and flu germs. These nutrients, in conjunction with 1 g of vitamin C every day, will help to promote your general health and well-being, and before long those stressful experiences will become exciting challenges.

We must all remember that both the good in our lives and the disease are the results of thought patterns which we form from our experiences. Thoughts are living things – everything begins with a thought. We all have positive and negative thoughts – the positive ones produce good, productive actions, while the negative ones produce only uncomfortable and unrewarding experiences. The important thing is that you are what you think. Think only good thoughts, healthy thoughts, loving, flexible thoughts, be calm and peaceful, and the health of your mind will return, along with the health of your body. You will experience love, joy, and contentment in your life and in all your surroundings, and in those you come into contact with day by day. Remember the old adage, 'As you think, so you are'. Think healthy – you will be healthy, think lucky – you will be lucky.

Thank your for reading this book – I hope you will benefit from it.

Index

Acid-free diet 75
Adenoids 35–8, 49, 52
Alcohol 22–3, 28, 90, 107
Antibiotics 2, 29, 37, 64–5,
    94

Bedsores 93
Bread 21
Bronchitis 48, 53, 73, 98

Calcium 102–3, 106
Carbohydrates 18–20, 21
Children 7, 12, 38–42, 67–76
Cider vinegar 36, 55
Clothing
    for children 70
    for older people 84
Coffee 22
Colds 35–46, 97, 101
    treating colds 42–46
Constipation 25, 49, 80–82,
    101
Convalescence 90–93
Croup 50
Cough mixture 52
Coughs 47–59 *and*
    throughout
    treating coughs 51–59

Deafness 36, 71

Depression 86, 101
Diarrhoea 49, 101
Diet 15–26, 36, 82–3
    for children 38–42
Digestion 18–20
Diphtheria 36
Disinfectants 44–5
Drugs 1–4

Enemas 25, 63–4, 83
Epidemics 60
Exercise 12, 32–3, 67, 72,
    78, 86, 106
Eyesight 71, 84–5
Eyestrain 85

Fasting 16–17, 55, 57, 63,
    83, 86
Fats 18–20, 21
Fevers 45–6
Fibre 21, 25, 80–81, 82
Flu 2, 13, 54, 60 *and*
    throughout
Food 15–26, 69–70

Gargles 43

Hair 70
Hearing 71, 85
Heart disease 49

Honey 36
Hypochondria 14

Incubation period 62
Indigestion 31, 49, 98, 101
Insomnia 31

Kidneys 28–9, 31, 78

Laryngitis 53, 58
Lungs 28, 78

Menus 23–5
Middle age 5, 12, 95
Midlife crisis 95
Migraine 74–5, 101
Minerals 23–5
Multivitamins 25, 93, 99–100

Nervous cough 50
Nursing 88–93
Nutrition 12, 13

Old age 5, 12, 87–88
Osteoporosis 101–3
Overeating 17

Prevention 14
Proteins 18–20, 21, 29

Quinsy 56

Scarlet fever 54, 57

Shock 13
Side-effects 1
Skin 27–8, 78
Sleep 12, 30–32, 41, 72–3
Smokers' cough 50
Smoking 23, 32, 33–4, 37,
    39, 85, 98, 105–6
Sore throat 53–6
Steroids 1
Stomach 31
Stomach cough 45–50
Stress 86, 101, 104–6
Suppression 2, 3

Tea 22
Teeth 71–2
Tonsilitis 36, 38, 54, 56, 57
Tonsils 35–7, 49, 52
Toxic acids 2, 3

Valium 105, 107
Vegetarians 21–2
Vincent's angina 54, 57
Vitamins 94–103
    A 96, 97, 99, 100–101
    B 96, 97, 99, 101, 106
    C 43, 56, 57, 66, 96, 97–9,
      106
    D 96, 97, 99, 100–101, 102
    E 99, 101–2

Water 21, 22, 25, 70, 90
Whooping cough 48–9
Women 12, 86, 103, 104–5

The Margaret Hills Series

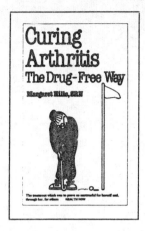

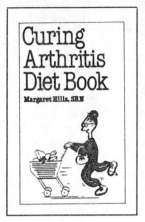

Bestselling advice for everyday problems, to help you take the first step to a healthier life.

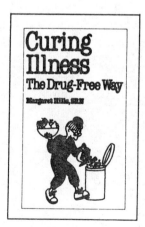

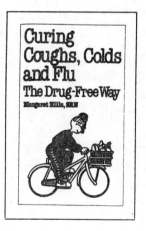